OXFORD MEDICAL PUF

Autism

THE FACTS

Autism

THE FACTS

SIMON BARON-COHEN
*The Institute of Psychiatry,
University of London*

and PATRICK BOLTON
*Department of Child Psychiatry,
University of Cambridge*

Oxford New York Tokyo
OXFORD UNIVERSITY PRESS

Oxford University Press, Great Clarendon Street, Oxford OX2 6DP

Oxford New York
Athens Auckland Bangkok Bogota Bombay
Buenos Aires Calcutta Cape Town Dar es Salaam
Delhi Florence Hong Kong Istanbul Karachi
Kuala Lumpur Madras Madrid Melbourne
Mexico City Nairobi Paris Singapore
Taipei Tokyo Toronto
and associated companies in
Berlin Ibadan

Oxford is a trade mark of Oxford University Press

Published in the United States by
Oxford University Press Inc., New York

First published 1993
Reprinted 1993 (twice), 1994, 1995, 1996 (twice)

A catalogue record for this book is available from the British Library

Library of Congress Cataloging in Publication Data
Autism : the facts / Simon Baron-Cohen and Patrick Bolton.
(Oxford medical publications) (The Facts)
Includes bibliographical references and index.
1. Autism in children—Popular works. I. Bolton, Patrick.
II. Title. III. Series. IV. Series: Facts/OPB.
[DNLM: 1. Autism—popular works. WM 203.5 B265a]
RJ506.A9B28 1993 618.92'8982—dc20 92–49828
ISBN 0 19 262327 3 (pbk.)

Printed and bound in Great Britain by
Biddles Ltd, Guildford and King's Lynn

Preface

As scientists carrying out research into autism, we were asked to write a book for parents, explaining what is known about autism, from the scientific point of view. This book is our attempt to do just that, and is written first and foremost for families of children with autism. However, we hope that it will also be useful for health professionals and others looking for a straightforward introduction to autism. Parents and others need easy access to the scientific facts, and our aim in writing this book has been to put these into a digestible form.

Throughout the book we avoid academic references in the text, so as not to deter the non-academic reader. We decided on a question-and-answer format, where appropriate, because parents are often looking for answers to key questions about autism. Examples of such questions include *What happens to children with autism when they grow up? Does autism run in families?* and *What kind of educational setting is best?* In collaboration with the National Autistic Society, who receive literally thousands of such questions every year via their telephone advice-line and regional conferences, from parents and professionals alike, we have been able to discover which questions are most on people's minds, and have attempted to answer these.

This book does not take a dogmatic approach to autism. Rather, our aim is to lay the scientific facts out in front of you, so that the complexities of autism cease to be so fragmented, and so that you can make your own decisions from an informed position about your child.

A note about terminology
In line with current thinking in the field of disability, we have taken seriously the issue of avoiding terms that may be offensive. In particular, we follow the recent practice of labelling the disability, rather than the person, and agree that this is both more accurate and more humane. This book is therefore about 'children with autism', and not 'autistic children', or 'autistics'. In addition, we use the term 'children with autism' only when we are specifically talking about *children* with this disability, and not adolescents or adults.

Terminology is often difficult to get right, and we certainly would not claim to have achieved complete success at this. Thus, we opt to use the term 'autism' even though some would argue that such labels are harmful in themselves. We disagree with this view, believing that if a person has this disability, the clear identification of this should also mean better access to educational and other benefits. Naturally we share the conviction that if a label is leading to negative effects, such as institutionalization or a loss of hope, this is wrong. But we hope that with better information and public resources, labels such as these will only have positive effects.

We have included a Glossary at the end of the book, to define more technical terms and phrases. In addition, at the end of the book you will find an Appendix that lists the international agencies of relevance to autism.

London   S.B.-C.
September 1992   P.B.

Acknowledgements

In writing this book we have been helped by many people. We would like to thank Tessa Hall, Mark Bebbington, Christine Nickles, Geraldine Peacock, Julie Hoare, Lorna Wing, Amita Shah, Pat Howlin, Ellen Heptinstall, Rita Jordan, and Colin Bolton. All these people read drafts of the book, and their valuable comments helped us to improve it. A special acknowledgement is owed to Bridget Lindley, who patiently reworked the detail of the text to make it more reader-friendly. We have also benefited from discussions with a large number of colleagues on issues in this book, particularly Mick Connolly, Phil Christie, Donald Cohen, Helen Tager-Flusberg, June Felton, Uta Frith, and Michael Rutter.

We are grateful to the following for providing illustrations: The Charing Cross Hospital Medical Illustration Department, for Figs. 2, 3, and 4; Professor Eric Courchesne, for Fig. 5; *Cognition*, for Fig. 7; The Walt Disney Company, London, for Fig. 8; Academic Press Inc. London, for Figs. 9 and 10; J. M. Dent and Sons Ltd, for Figs. 11 and 12; Dr Rita Jordan, for Fig. 16; and finally, Christine Nickles and the National Autistic Society for Figs. 6, 13, 14, 15, 17, and 18. Appendix 2 has been reproduced with the permission of the American Psychiatric Association and the World Health Organization.

This book is dedicated to those children with autism and their families who have helped us for many years in our research. We are pleased to be able to offer you something in return.

Contents

1.

Introducing two children with autism

Autism is a condition that affects some children from either birth or infancy, and leaves them unable to form normal social relationships, or to develop normal communication. As a result, the child may become isolated from human contact and absorbed in a world of repetitive, obsessional activities and interests.

Children with autism may behave in strange ways. They may jump up and down excitedly at the sight of the water running from the taps, yet ignore attempts by adults to turn activities into a 'social' game in which others can share. They may look past you, or only very briefly at you, and make you feel as if you are an unimportant part of their world. They may call you when they need something, but otherwise virtually ignore you, spending hours lining up objects in the living room, or flapping their hands and fingers excitedly as they repeatedly flick through picture books or magazines.

In most of the chapters in this book we will be focusing on what is known about autism, and on the needs of children and adults with the condition. In this opening chapter however, we introduce you to two typical children that we might expect to see in our clinic. They would both be diagnosed as having autism, though in one case it is severe, while in the other it is less so. The details of these cases are compilations of several children we have known, in order to bring out a range of features.

John

John, an only child, was born after a normal pregnancy and delivery. As an infant, he was easy to breast-feed, the transition to solid foods posed no difficulties, and he also slept well. At first, his mother and father were delighted at how easy he was: he seemed happy and content to lie in his cot for hours. He sat unsupported at six months (which is within the normal range), and soon after he crawled energetically. His parents considered him to be independent and wilful. However, his grandmother was puzzled by his independence. To her mind, he showed an undue preference for his own company: it was as if he lacked interest in people.

John walked on his first birthday, much to the delight of his parents; yet during his second year he did not progress as well as expected. Although he made sounds, he did not use words. Indeed, his ability to communicate was so limited that even when he was three years old his mother still found herself trying to guess what he wanted (much as if he were a far younger child). Often she tried giving him a drink or some food in the hope that she had guessed his needs correctly. Occasionally he would grab hold of her wrist and drag her over to the sink, yet he never said anything like 'drink', or pointed to the tap.

This was obviously a source of concern in itself; but at about this time his parents also became concerned about his extreme independence. For example, even when he fell down, he would not come to his parents to show them he had hurt himself. At times they even felt he was uninterested in them, because he never became upset when his mother had to go out and leave him with a neighbour or relative. In fact, he seemed to be more interested in playing with his bricks than in spending time with people. He made long straight lines of bricks over and over again. He spent an extraordinary number of hours lining them up in exactly the same way and in precisely the same sequence of colours.

From time to time, his parents also worried about his hearing and wondered if he were deaf, particularly as he often showed no response when they called his name. At other times, however, his hearing seemed to be very acute: he would turn his head at the slightest sound of a plane going over the house, or of a fire-engine siren in the distance. In the weeks following his third birthday they became increasingly concerned, despite reassurances from the health professionals. He was not using any words to express himself, and he showed no interest in playing with other children. For example, he did not wave *bye-bye* or show any real joy when they tried to play *peek-a-boo*. His mother agonized about her relationship with John, because he always wriggled away from her cuddles, and only seemed to like rough-and-tumble play with his father. She worried that she had done something wrong as a mother, and felt depressed, rejected, and guilty.

When he was three and a half years old the GP referred John to a specialist. The specialist, a child psychiatrist, told the parents that John had autism, but added that his psychological abilities in spatial tasks (such as jigsaw puzzles) suggested that his intellectual abilities were normal in these areas. The specialist thought it was too early to give an accurate picture of the way he would progress, but said there were some indications to suggest he would do better than most children with autism. John was sent to a special playgroup, and received speech therapy. A psychologist visited the family at home and helped the parents plan ways of encouraging the development of communication, and reducing the frequency of his temper tantrums.

In his fourth year, John suddenly began to speak in complete sentences. His parents were greatly relieved, and for a time actually believed he had finally 'grown out' of the problems. However, his speech was quite unusual. For example, he often repeated back word for word whatever his parents had said. So, if they asked him 'Do you want a drink?', he would say 'You want a drink' in reply. At other times, John made rather surprising remarks. For instance, he would say 'You really tickle me' in a tone of voice exactly similar to that of a family friend who had first used the expression some days before. However, his use of this phrase, and most of his speech, was usually inappropriate to the setting, and lacked any clear meaning.

The years from four to six were very difficult for the family. Despite speech therapy and special help at school, John only made slow progress. He developed a fascination with vacuum cleaners and lampposts, and started to draw them over and over again. He became exceptionally excited whenever his mother took out the vacuum cleaner, jumping up and down and vigorously flapping his arms and flicking his fingers near his eyes. He also became preoccupied by lights, rushing around the house switching them on and off. Even family outings became an ordeal: John threw wild tantrums unless the family took exactly the same route and let him count all the lampposts. He never seemed to tire of doing exactly the same thing over and over again.

His behaviour was also unusual in other ways, in that he never really seemed to look at anyone directly. Rather, he would look at them only fleetingly or else not at all. Despite this, John seemed to notice everything in minute detail. He could ride his bicycle along the most crowded pavements without knocking anyone over, and he spotted car number-plates with a figure four in them long before anyone else had noticed. He would also do things his parents found embarrassing, like grabbing and eating sandwiches from a stranger's plate at restaurants. As a consequence, they had to stop going to restaurants.

When John started school, he found it difficult to learn to read and write, although in other areas of work he was very quick. For example, he was very good with his number work, and took a great delight in learning multiplication tables. He was also still very quick at jigsaws, and could manage even difficult puzzles quite easily: at six years old, he did a 200-piece jigsaw puzzle on his own, and a 100-piece one upside-down! Socially, however, he was unable to make any friends whatsoever. He would attempt to join in a game that he liked, but his approaches were so odd that other children tended to ignore him. Most of the time, John was to be found on his own, busying himself with one of his special interests, more absorbed in counting lampposts than in playing with other school-children.

From the age of seven, John was sent to a special school for children with autism. At about this age his parents also noticed that he seemed more interested in their company. He would, for example, show his mother he had hurt himself when he fell down, and he even seemed to derive some comfort and pleasure from cuddles. Also, he began to wait for his father to come home from work, and even started to look out for him. However, his parents were never sure whether John truly enjoyed seeing his father return, or whether he was simply waiting to see if his father came home at exactly six o'clock.

Fortunately, while at school he developed more and more. He is now nineteen years old, and no longer simply repeats things he has heard, but is able to make appropriate comments and hold a simple conversation about a topic of interest. Similarly, he is able to read simple books, although he has difficulty grasping the story-line. However, he has very little interest in either reading or conversing. Instead he prefers to pursue his current interest in collecting bottle-tops and listening to pop music. He watches all the TV programmes about pop music, and seems to derive enormous pleasure from writing out, or reciting, a list of all the current hit records and their order in the charts. He has learnt all these lists by heart, and can tell you what the top twenty records were on any particular date for many years back.

Although he has mastered simple social pleasantries, he still finds social gatherings very difficult, and always ends up on the periphery of any group. He has not established any close friendships, despite his desire to do so. Sadly, this troubles him. Recently he asked his parents how to make friends. They found it hard to explain what to most people comes naturally.

Currently, John has a place in sheltered employment, fitting com-ponents into radios. He is considered to be a reliable and careful worker. However, his employers feel unable to allocate more responsibility to him because he seems unable to master the social skills required for dealing with colleagues and customers. He has some awareness of these problems, and talks about his difficulty in understanding other people. 'I never know what they are going to do next', he says. Yet despite this insight, he has unrealistic expectations about the future. In particular, he expects to marry and have a family, but seems to have no firm grasp of what this might entail.

Lucy

Lucy is the second child in her family. She has a brother, Mark, who is four years older. Lucy's parents kept an eye on her development right from the start, because there had been so many difficulties during the pregnancy and delivery. To begin with, there had been a slight show of blood in the 14th week; and later the obstetrician had become concerned about Lucy's rate of growth in the womb. On the ultrasound scan, Lucy's mother and father were so excited to see their baby moving about that it came as a hard blow when they were told the baby was 'small for dates'. Labour commenced three weeks early, and lasted 23 hours, so that eventually forceps were needed to assist the delivery. Immediately after the birth there were further problems: Lucy had to have oxygen to revive her, and she had to spend four days in the special-care baby-unit, and to receive ultraviolet-light treatment for jaundice. Understandably, Lucy's parents felt she was 'delicate' right from the start.

Indeed, it seemed that, in comparison to her brother, everything in Lucy's development was a source of concern. Feeding Lucy was one of the problems. When her mother tried to breast-feed her, she either seemed too distressed to feed or else she fed so ravenously and quickly that minutes later she would vomit. Lucy's mother doesn't remember a single 'easy' feed. Nights were no better, as Lucy took hours to settle, and always woke early. The feeding and sleeping difficulties continued for years with little improvement.

By Lucy's first birthday there was cause for more concern. She had only just started to sit up, and she was still not crawling. Everyone else's baby seemed to be at the stage of pulling themselves up on the furniture, and some had even taken their first steps. The parents consulted their GP, who told them that Lucy was indeed delayed in her development, and that at this stage it was best to keep an eye on how she progressed.

At 14 months Lucy started to crawl, and at 19 months she pulled herself up on the furniture; but she seemed to make little progress in other areas of development.

At two years old Lucy was still not using any words, and was unresponsive to her parents' attempts to engage her in even simple games like *peek-a-boo* and *round-and-round-the-garden*. She was seen by a paediatrician, who told the parents that the delay in her development might be due to the difficulties with the delivery at her birth. It was suggested that Lucy should attend the clinic every 12 months for a regular review.

By 30 months Lucy had started to walk, much to the relief of her parents. However, she was still not making any meaningful sounds—indeed, her main sounds were a strange clicking noise she made with the back of her tongue, and a variety of screams. Her parents were exasperated, and bitterly envied the obvious pleasure other parents seemed to get from *their* children. Moreover, Lucy still seemed oblivious to people around her (including her parents) unless they had something she wanted. For example, she loved to play with a particular blue and red rattle. If anyone took this out, Lucy would run over and leap on that person, staring directly into their eyes with her face very close, and then grab the rattle and run off to a corner of the room. There she would shake it or spin it round and round. Once she had the rattle, she did not bother to look at anyone, or offer it to others. If someone tried to take the rattle from her, she would scream and bang her head on the floor. Understandably, this devastated her parents. To prevent the head-banging, they endeavoured to ensure that other people never touched the rattle. Gradually, they began to feel that their lives were totally controlled by Lucy.

Lucy showed other odd behaviour. For example, she took great interest in the smell of everything, sniffing food, toys, clothes, and (to her parents' embarrassment) people. She even tried to smell strangers in the street. She also liked the touch and feel of things—especially sandpaper. In fact, she insisted on carrying around a small piece of sandpaper in her pocket. Strangely, though, she took no interest in the cuddly toys she was given. Lucy's desire to touch and feel things was also a source of embarrassment to her parents. She often tried to stroke stockings on women's legs, even if they were complete strangers. If they tried to stop her, she would have a tantrum.

When Lucy turned four years old, the paediatrician said she suspected Lucy suffered from autism, and suggested the family should attend a child psychiatric centre for a detailed assessment. Following the appointment, the diagnosis was confirmed; but in addition, her parents were told that Lucy was generally delayed in her development. They were heartbroken at the news of her diagnosis, because it seemed so permanent. Nevertheless, they also felt some relief at having a diagnosis, after four years of not knowing what was wrong. They felt that finally Lucy would get the help she desperately needed. Following the assessment, Lucy was sent to a special playgroup for children with mental handicap, and speech and music therapy were started. At the same time, the parents were put in touch with the National Autistic Society, to help them obtain local support from other parents.

Over the next year the temper tantrums stopped, following treatments by a psychologist, and life for the family became a little more manageable. Nevertheless, Lucy continued to behave unusually. She never paid any attention to the arrivals and departures of her parents or friends, unless it was to try to sniff them. She would run around the house in a strict systematic order and check the position of little pieces of cotton she had tied to all the chairs. If any of these were even fractionally out of place, she would immediately reposition them. Similarly, if one of these was missing she became inconsolable until it was found or replaced. Also, Lucy became very upset whenever she heard the sound of a motorbike. In these situations she would whimper and cover her ears with her hands. Strangely, other sounds seemed to be a source of fascination. For example, she loved to listen to the washing-machine, and when it was on she would shriek with delight and press her ear to the machine until the washing cycle finished.

At the age of six, Lucy moved to a special school for children with autism. Initially this was as a day pupil, but when she was ten it was suggested she become a weekly boarder so as to relieve the strain on her parents. At school and under supervision, she learned to wash, dress, and feed herself, and she also learned to cut out shapes with a pair of scissors. However, she never learned to read, write, or speak, although she enjoyed looking through picture-books.

Her favourite activity was, and still is, watching cartoons on television: in fact, when her parents purchased a video recorder she learned how to play videos of cartoons. Usually she replays the same tape over and over again, always showing great delight when characters trip and fall. When excited she flaps her arms, rises up on tiptoe, and bites her hand. An imaginative teacher at school taught Lucy to keep her hands in her pockets, and this simple strategy has prevented much of her hand-biting.

She knows that she can take her hands out of her pockets to use them for sign-language, which she is slowly learning, and then put them back into her pockets again.

At fourteen, Lucy developed epilepsy. Fortunately, this was success-fully treated with medication. Five years later, having reached the end of school, she moved to a sheltered residential unit for adults with autism, and here she developed her fondness for horse-riding and cooking, interests which had begun in the final years at school. She visits her family regularly, yet she does not seem to show much interest in seeing her old schoolfriends. Instead, she prefers to spend her time looking through old magazines, alone in her bedroom, or walking in the park behind the hostel.

She has not made any new friends as such, nor has she developed any speech, although she has learnt about fifty simple signs to indicate, for example, that she wishes to use the toilet, or that she would like a toy, food, or drink, or to go to the park. At times there have been periods when Lucy has again injured herself by head-banging. Thankfully, this self-injury is no longer a problem. However, she does have episodes when she pulls out her own hair. Keeping her hands in her pockets is still a solution for this.

Why are John and Lucy so different?

John and Lucy share the characteristic problems of autism: they both failed to develop normal social relationships and communication in the first three years of life, and both of them showed unusual interests and repetitive preoccupations.

Lucy is typical of some children with autism in being very unrespons-ive—so unresponsive that when she was young her parents described her as 'living in a glass bubble' or being 'locked in a private world'. By contrast, John is typical of another group of children with autism in that he is quite outgoing socially, approaches others in a talkative and self-confident manner, and often asks them quite precise and factual ques-tions. For example, he asks all new visitors to his school '*Why do people wear glasses? Which bus do you take to work?*'. However, John's attempts at social interaction are still repetitive and stilted. So John's communication abnormalities are rather subtle, and consist of speaking in this one-sided, repetitive way; whereas Lucy lacks almost any ability to communicate.

In addition to these problems in social and language development, both John and Lucy show 'classic' ritualistic behaviour: doing the same activity over and over again in an identical fashion. For example, Lucy checks the position of her little threads tied on all the chairs in the house, whereas John insists on taking exactly the same route to school each day. They also have very repetitive interests. John, for example, likes nothing better than counting lampposts, while Lucy will watch the same video many times in one day, if she is allowed. They can spend hours immersed in nothing but these narrow interests. These 'obsessions' sometimes lead to problems. For example, when he was young, John often screamed intensely and inconsolably if a piece of a puzzle was missing, or if a change occurred in his daily routine. As an adult, he still finds change difficult to cope with.

Thus, despite the similarities between John and Lucy, these two children illustrate how abnormal behaviour in autism can vary. These differences are due to three key factors:

● *Mental handicap*

Autism is frequently (but not always) associated with mental handicap. Lucy has both autism and mental handicap, while John just has autism. This meant that all aspects of Lucy's development were slower to emerge, and her overall level of functioning was quite limited; her interests are more restricted than John's. (In the UK and in some other countries, the term *learning difficulties* is sometimes used instead of *mental handicap*.)

● *Language level*

The severity of language problems in autism can also vary markedly. Thus John has really quite a lot of speech, whereas Lucy is virtually mute. Naturally, many children with autism fall somewhere in between these two extremes. The amount of language a child acquires strongly affects the range of opportunities available for that child, as well as other aspects of development, and consequently influences how autism is manifested.

● *Age*

As children with autism grow older, so the pattern of autism changes. For example, with age some become more outgoing, and others develop speech, while yet others seem to make little progress. Substantial gains are usually only seen in those children who do not have additional mental handicap, and in those with well-developed speech.

If your child has autism, then it is important to ask the specialist the extent to which your child has additional disabilities such as mental handicap or language disorder. This information is essential in planning realistically for his or her future, and will affect the kind of school to be chosen. Naturally, the two contrasting examples of John and Lucy represent extremes, and many children with autism will have milder handicaps than Lucy shows.

Some common questions about autism

What causes autism?

Thirty years ago autism was thought to result from poor parenting. This view turned out to be factually wrong. Parents of children with autism are as loving and caring and competent as any other parents. Tragically, however, this early view caused untold upset: parents not only had to cope with their child's autism, but also with the guilt of believing they were the cause. Modern medical evidence suggests clear biological causes for autism, and this has meant that parents no longer need to blame themselves. The suggested biological causes include genetic factors, viral infections, and birth or pregnancy complications, any of which may cause the subtle brain damage assumed to produce autism. These biological causes are not found in every child with autism, which suggests that other biological factors are still to be discovered. The biology of autism is discussed in Chapters 4 and 5.

Will my next child have autism?

Parents naturally worry, after their child starts to show autism, whether they might have passed this on through their genes. This then raises a further worry for some parents as to whether they should go on to have other children. This is a difficult question to give answers to. We know that the risks of autism are increased in some families; but clear-cut advice regarding the extent of risk for individual families is not possible at present. Parents who are concerned about this issue may like to discuss it with a genetic counsellor. The National Autistic Society can provide information on how to be referred for genetic counselling in your area. Thankfully, most parents with a child with autism do go on to have other healthy, normal children. The possible role of genetics in autism is discussed in Chapter 4.

Do children with autism come from any particular family background?

Leo Kanner, the psychiatrist who first described autism (in 1943) observed that many of the children with autism seen in his clinic came from well-educated, intelligent parents from the middle and upper social classes. However, it appears that as the services for the diagnosis of autism have become more widely available, so it has been found equally in all social classes. Similarly, autism occurs in all cultures, so far as is known. Surveys from a range of different countries have consistently reported that between 2 and 4 children in every 10 000 develop autism, usually in the ratio of 3–4 boys to each girl. The similarity between these studies, despite very different locations and methods of data collection, suggests that the biological causes of autism are largely independent of cultural factors. If broader criteria are used, the rate of autism may be as high as 15–20 per 10 000. Using such a figure, the National Autistic Society estimates that in the UK there may be as many as 85 000 people with autism or an autistic-like condition. The equivalent estimate from the Autism Society of America is between 300 000 and 400 000 individuals in the USA. The diagnosis of autism is described in Chapter 2.

Are children with autism of normal intelligence?

One widely held view is that children with autism are of normal intelligence but are simply unable to communicate this to other people because of their social and communication difficulties. As was evident from our description of Lucy, such a view does not fit many real cases. Indeed, when children with autism are given intelligence (IQ) tests, roughly two-thirds of them score in the below-average range. That is to say, like Lucy, they have mental handicap as well as autism. The remaining third have an IQ in the normal range. So autism can occur at any point on the intelligence spectrum. We look at the unusual aspects of intelligence and psychology in autism in Chapters 6 and 7.

Can children with autism be educated?

It used to be thought that children with autism were ineducable. Today, this view has thankfully been disproved, and governments in many countries now make provision for the special education of children with autism. Although there is still a serious shortage of places in special schools and units, it is essential to try to get your child into a school that understands autism. In the right setting, considerable progress can be made, as is described in Chapter 8.

What happens to these children when they grow up?

Autism is often thought to be a condition of childhood alone, probably because so much is said about *children* with autism. But what happens to such children when they become adults? Do they have a shorter life expectancy? Is that why one hears so little about adults with autism? Or do they grow out of the autism? The answer is that most children do not grow out of autism when they reach adulthood, nor do they have a shorter life expectancy than other people with comparable handicaps, as far as is known. Until recently, parents' organizations put all their energies into pressurizing government agencies into providing services for children with autism, since this was clearly the highest priority. This may explain why we do not hear as much about adults with autism. Priorities have shifted recently, with campaigns for appropriate provision for adults too. In addition, since the disorder itself was only recognized in 1943, it is only in recent years that people diagnosed as having autism in childhood have reached adulthood. The special needs of adults with autism are discussed in Chapter 11.

Can people recover from autism?

As was stated above, autism tends to persist into adulthood. This sounds pessimistic, implying that there is no chance of recovery. There are a few isolated claims of recovery from autism, but these reports do not give details of how full a recovery has been made. For example, some reports claim a recovery if the person starts to talk, or to smile and show affection, or to learn. But, as we shall see, these are not by themselves signs of a complete recovery. They do reflect improvements, but usually autism continues throughout life. Treatments for autism are still rather limited in what they can achieve. The range of treatments available is discussed in Chapters 8 to 10.

Can allergies or food additives cause autism?

Recent publicity has focused on the role of foods and allergies in illness. The scientific evidence currently suggests that, in a few children who have problems with *hyperactivity*, dietary additives and preservatives may play some part in their problems. At the present time, however, there is scant evidence to indicate that allergies or dietary factors can actually cause autism, or that they affect the social and communication problems. They may affect the child's level of activity and ability to concentrate, however. The role of diet in treatment is discussed in Chapter 10.

In the next chapter, we turn to one of the very first questions faced by parents who suspect their child may have autism: how is the diagnosis made?

2.

How the diagnosis is made

Long before we even got to the clinic my wife and I knew that John had autism. It was just obvious he was not the same as other kids. But we still needed to hear it from them. That was because we still hoped we might be wrong. On the other hand, we were desperate to get some hard facts to use as evidence in our fight with the school system, to make sure John got what was best for him.

Diagnosis is essential if different conditions are to be clearly distinguished, with a view to both understanding and treating different disorders. Early diagnosis offers the hope that treatment can start before the condition has pushed the child too far off the normal course of development. At present, early diagnosis of autism is still rare; but doctors are currently working towards improving the diagnostic tools to achieve this goal. In this chapter, we describe an assessment format used in Britain, pointing out how autism is distinguished from superficially similar conditions. We also discuss the consequences of diagnosis.

How is the diagnosis made?

Autism is a behavioural syndrome, meaning there is a *cluster* of abnormal types of behaviour. The diagnosis of autism is only made if this cluster of three key types of behaviour is present. The key behaviours are:

- The child's social relationships and social development are abnormal.
- The child is failing to develop normal communication.
- The child's interests and activities are restricted and repetitive, rather than flexible and imaginative.

It is worth stressing that a diagnosis of autism would not be made merely because a child has problems in language *or* social interaction *or* imagination, but only if these types of behaviour all occur *together*, signifying the distinct pattern of autism. Naturally, in defining autism in this way, it is crucial to understand what is meant by *normal* development. This in itself is complex, and therefore the diagnosis can only really be done by experts who have considerable experience in recognizing both normal and abnormal child development.

There is one final factor which is considered in making the diagnosis. This is the *age* at which the symptoms were first identified. The World Health Organization's system for classifying medical disorders (called ICD-10) requires that all three symptoms must have been present by 36 months of age; the American system (called DSM-IIIR) also requires that the age of onset should be recorded. The full set of criteria for diagnosing autism under these two systems are shown in Appendix 2.

The assessment

There are a number of different approaches to assessing children with developmental problems. However, the basic principles are usually the same at each centre.

Part of the assessment must take place at a clinic, because the procedure often involves a variety of specialist investigations, such as intelligence and language testing, and medical and neurological examinations. The clinic setting also provides a 'standardized' context for observing the nature of the child's difficulties. Although parents may be exasperated by the apparently uncharacteristic behaviour of their child in this setting, it nevertheless provides a way of comparing one child with others. But the clinic-based assessment is only one part of the whole assessment. If necessary, the picture is further built up by observing the child at home and at the school or nursery, during play, and in situations in which natural communication and social interaction should be occurring. The clinic assessment often takes the best part of a day visit, during which the team (usually a child psychiatrist, a clinical or educational psychologist, and a psychiatric social worker) observe the child and discuss their findings. This process is lengthy simply because autism can be confused with other conditions.

Distinguishing autism from other conditions

Often, the task for the clinician is to decide whether the child has autism or some other, similar condition. Autism can, at first glance, be confused with a number of conditions. It may, for example, appear similar to *elective mutism* (a condition in which the child simply refuses to talk in certain situations) or to *attachment disorder* (where a child fails to

develop stable emotional bonds with his or her parents, possibly following abuse, deprivation, or family problems). Autism is also superficially
similar to *specific language disorder* (where language is delayed, but
where social development may be relatively normal). Finally, various
kinds of *mental handicap* (where all skills are delayed, social ones
included) can sometimes resemble autism. All of these alternative
diagnoses need to be firmly ruled out before a child is finally given the
diagnosis of autism.

One final complication in the diagnosis of autism is that an autism-like
pattern may appear, but with one or more of the features missing. This is
seen in *atypical autism* (where only one or two autistic features are
present, and where these features may not necessarily appear before
three years of age). It is also found in *Asperger's syndrome* (where
intelligence and early language development may be fairly normal, but
where the social abnormalities are still present). Parents may then be told
that their child does not have classic autism, but simply has 'autistic
features'. This is a frustrating term, in that it leaves parents unclear
whether their child does or does not have autism. But this situation
reflects the fact that there are some grey areas between clearly having the
condition and not having it. Sometimes, development is abnormal in all
three key areas, but the picture does not quite resemble classic autism.
In these circumstances, a diagnosis of *other pervasive developmental
disorder* is given.

Other conditions, such as *Rett's syndrome* (in which girls show neurological problems such as hand-wringing and other odd hand movements),
and *disintegrative disorder* (in which the child rapidly deteriorates in all
skills, after a period of normal development) may be similar to autism, so
careful assessment is essential. The same applies to conditions such as
hyperkinetic disorder with stereotypies (in which children suffer from
very poor concentration, clumsiness, restlessness and repetitive behaviour), and *Landau–Kleffner syndrome* (a condition characterized by a
period of normal language development followed by a fluctuating loss of
speech and accompanied by epilepsy). Table 2.1 lists these alternative
diagnoses.

Other conditions and behavioural problems

To complicate matters further, some children can end up receiving more
than one diagnosis. The additional problems that are sometimes seen
include anxiety, self-injury (such as head-banging and hand-biting),

toilet-training difficulties, hyperactivity (excessive restlessness and fidgeting), and Gilles de la Tourette's syndrome (multiple tics, with involuntary vocalizations). Most of these other conditions are fortunately quite rare in people with autism. But in the overall diagnosis these may need to be assessed too, so that when giving advice about treatment, these additional difficulties can be helped. Parents should feel able to ask their doctor exactly what the diagnosis means for their child.

Table 2.1: Conditions with similarities to autism

- *Elective mutism*
- *Attachment disorder*
- *Developmental receptive language disorder*
- *Hyperkinetic disorder with stereotypies*
- *Disintegrative disorder*
- *Mental handicap*
- *Rett's syndrome*
- *Landau–Kleffner syndrome*

Immediate consequences of diagnosis

If your child does fit the picture of autism, it may seem that your worst fears have come true. Secretly you may have been hoping to hear that the problems were only mild and would pass. The diagnosis may then be a terrible shock. Consider, for example, how one parent expressed the feelings she experienced after diagnosis:

. . . the paediatrician came to see me. He asked me if I actually had any idea what was wrong with my son. I replied that my father-in-law and one of my friends had both suggested that he might be mildly autistic, though I myself had no real idea what the word meant. He nodded. 'I am afraid they are right', he told me, very gently. 'Simon is autistic. I am afraid that you have a long, hard road ahead of you.' . . . I looked at him. Nothing seemed real any more. He was certainly not real. It was as if he had just fallen to pieces in front of my eyes . . . Everything—my way of life, my pride, my confidence, my whole outlook—had just been totally and irrevocably shattered. The numbness was merciful. It was better that I should realize slowly how much we, but above all, Simon, had lost (Ann Lovell, *In a Summer Garment*, Secker and Warburg, London, 1978, p. 18).

The different stages in the reaction to the diagnosis are considered in more detail in the next chapter. Whatever the response, parents often feel apprehension about the future and confused about the condition. Any diagnostic assessment should be followed by sensitive discussion with the family about the nature of their child's problems, their severity, and the expected future course. Further information and support should always be provided.

As we explained in the opening chapter, families are usually put in touch with the National Autistic Society in the UK, or its equivalent in other countries (these are listed in Appendix I). Such organizations provide additional advice, local parent-support groups, and information regarding recent developments in treatment and research. For the child, specific treatments and educational or nursery provisions are arranged depending on the nature of the problems and the age of the child. These are discussed in Chapters 7–9.

Why is autism not diagnosed in infancy?

As was mentioned earlier, autism usually becomes evident at some time in the first few years of life. The question then arises as to why it is not usually picked up in infancy. At present it is rare to diagnose the condition before the age of two years; and, in many instances, it is not diagnosed until considerably later.

There are a number of reasons for this. First, before two years of age, the pattern of behaviour may not be clear enough to allow a definitive diagnosis to be made. Secondly, when children with autism also have mental handicap, it may be the mental handicap which is the main cause for concern, and concentration on this may then allow the autism to go undetected. Thirdly, one of the main problems in autism involves speech and language. Consequently, diagnosis is much easier when development has progressed to an extent that allows for a full language assessment. Fourthly, in a few children with autism there is an initial period of relatively normal development, followed by the emergence of autism and a loss of skills. This decline may not occur until two years of age: obviously diagnosis in these circumstances is impossible before the problems begin.

In addition to these reasons, a late diagnosis may simply occur because parents who have no experience of the developmental milestones of normal children may not be aware of the problems in their child's development. After all, no parents like to think that their child has problems. The GP or health visitor may also have difficulties identifying the subtle difficulties of autism, and instead feel that they are either mild or transient developmental problems. This is not very surprising, given that it is unlikely for one of these health professionals to see even one case of autism during their whole career. As a consequence, parents are often told 'He'll grow out of it'. It is hoped that primary-health professionals will in time become better able to detect possible cases of autism and refer such cases on to specialists at younger ages, for suitable early intervention.

3.

Coping with the news

The diagnosis has helped clarify things for other people as much as for us, but the real struggle, of coming to terms with the fact that he'll never be normal and that the problems will never go away, will probably take us a lifetime to adjust to.

To discover your child suffers from a condition that results in some form of lifelong disability is, naturally, a tremendous blow. When parents finally realize that their child has autism, that it is not 'just a difficult phase he's going through', when they realize that in a sense they have 'lost' the child they thought they were going to have, they often feel overwhelmed by a wide range of emotions: sometimes despair and depression, coupled with anxiety about their child's future. At other times a cloak of guilt envelops them, at the thought of being in some way responsible for their child's condition. At yet other times, the emotion that takes over is a pervasive sense of shame or embarrassment, due to the imagined thoughts of others—'they've failed as parents'—which is of course untrue. All of these emotions are understandable reactions to the stresses and disappointments induced by the child's developmental problems. Faced with your child turning away from you, apparently more absorbed in some repetitive activity than in you, who wouldn't feel dismayed, rejected and frustrated?

Emotional reactions following the discovery of handicapping conditions

A fair amount is known about how parents respond to the discovery that their child has a disability. The following account is a description of the type of feelings that immediately follow when parents are told that their child has a handicapping condition like Down's Syndrome. We begin with this description because it best illustrates the range of feelings and thoughts that can occur in these circumstances. However, since autism is also different from all these other conditions, we follow this description with an outline of how the reaction following the discovery of autism may be different.

Not surprisingly, the immediate reactions are sometimes similar to those seen following bereavement: an initial phase of shock and disbelief (parents sometimes talk of feeling numb or cut off from the world). To some extent, the numbness helps prevent parents from being overwhelmed by their distress, and seems to act as a means of buffering them from the full significance of the discovery.

Understandably, parents find it difficult to assimilate new information during this stage, and may need to go through things several times, or at a later time, to grasp them fully. As a consequence, doctors should try to keep information short and simple when initially discussing the diagnosis, and then go through the details when parents have had a chance to recover from.hearing the news.

The early shock may be followed by a period of denial. Denial may be the mind's way of keeping anxiety and stress at bay. In its most pronounced form, it may result in people acting as if nothing has occurred; but usually it leads to parents minimizing the seriousness of the condition and fantasizing that their child will somehow be magically cured.

The next phase of the reaction is often full of feelings of anger and guilt. Anger at the injustice of the tragedy (How could this happen to me? What have I done to deserve this?), and guilt (What did we do to cause this?), turning to sadness and despair (How can we cope?). Finally, most parents adapt and become able to form a realistic picture of the problems, as well as of their child's strengths and special qualities, and begin to focus on practical ways of coping.

As has been explained, the above account is based on the reactions most often seen when the parents' discovery of the disability is sudden; on what typically occurs, for example, following the birth of children with a severe mental or physical handicap. The type of feelings parents experience following the diagnosis of autism may however be rather different. In the first place, since autism is not usually picked up until the child is at least two or three years of age, there may already have been concerns about the early development for some time before a specialist opinion is sought. As a consequence, many parents already suspect that something may be wrong, so that the news that their child has autism does not come as such a shock. Nevertheless, even when parents have suspected it, the final confirmation of the diagnosis can still come as a hard blow.

Other things may also affect the way in which parents react. For example, the severity of the autism and the degree of accompanying mental handicap may influence how you respond to the news. In addition, the psychological resilience of each parent, and the amount of support available from family, friends, and health professionals will also be important, helping some parents to pass through some stages more quickly than others.

In view of the fact that different individuals may pass through these stages at different rates or in different orders, it is important to recognize that members of the family who have not just heard the diagnosis may be at a different stage from those who have only just heard it, and that one's reactions may continue to be different from another's at any one time. They can help each other by showing their feelings. Couples may find it helpful to set aside regular times when they can discuss their worries, frustrations, and sadness together.

Extreme reactions

Sometimes individuals get 'stuck' in certain stages, or miss some out altogether, and this can lead to difficulties. Thus parents who continue to deny their child's handicap may embark on a relentless search for a cure, constantly seeking opinions from one specialist after another, never satisfied with the outcome. Continued searching for what might help the child is of course both important and valuable; but extreme reactions are often based more on the need to stave off the sad reality of their plight than on the child's needs. Yet other parents may get caught in an unresolved phase of anger, and become embroiled in protracted legal battles with professionals who they feel are responsible for the handicap. Again, valid legal redress is important; but extreme reactions are often based on the need to 'blame' someone. Distinguishing between normal and extreme reactions is not always straightforward.

The distress and feelings of sadness may also precipitate a severe depression. By depression in this context we mean not just feelings of ordinary sadness, but profound misery, together with an inability to derive pleasure from activities that are normally enjoyable. Often such depression also involves feelings of pessimism and worthlessness, as well as disturbed sleep and appetite. If this occurs, parents may benefit from professional help, either in the form of counselling, or antidepressant medication, or both. If this is a problem for you or your partner, you should ask your family doctor for help.

As we said earlier, most parents make a remarkable adaptation to their child's needs and problems. They come to realize that what they initially took as a *personal* rejection is simply the child's withdrawing because of not *understanding* the world in the same way as others do. Parents also come to realize that their child can respond affectionately to them after all—in his or her own way. The process of trying to understand their child's problems often brings with it a special intimacy, which comes from the feeling that this is a special child, who needs far more than most children, and with whom one does, in a unique way, develop a special relationship.

Effects on your marriage or relationship

Given the stresses of having a child with a handicap, it is small wonder that people often say that having a child with a disability makes or breaks a marriage. It may come as some reassurance, then, to learn that parents of children with autism are no more likely to separate and divorce than parents of non-handicapped children. Nevertheless, difficulties in the relationship may arise, and when this happens it is important to tackle them. Often no more is required than to set aside time for yourselves as partners (rather than just as parents) when you can talk openly, and share and discuss difficulties. To find time to do this may prove difficult; but the time is well worth the investment. If it proves difficult to arrange for friends or relatives to help with the child-care in order to give you some free time, then you should discuss this with one of the professionals involved with your child. There are facilities for family aid and respite care that have been developed just for this purpose which may be of value for you.

Effects on other children in your family

If you have other children, you will have to tell them of their brother's or sister's handicap. Precisely what is said will depend on the age of the particular child and their ability to grasp the problems. The news may also be a source of distress to them, and will need to be shared in a sensitive manner. It is also important to pace what you say, so that your child

is able to take the news on board and come to terms with it. It is not
enough to have a one-off 'heart to heart' talk and then leave it at that.
There will be a host of questions that your other child or children will
have about the problems and what they mean. It is essential that as
parents you discuss these issues openly and often, to avoid your child
'bottling up' their feelings and questions. Again, one way of avoiding
this difficulty is to provide times you can have alone with your other
child or children, when they know that they can ask you any questions
that are on their minds.

At present not much is known regarding the longer-term effects on
development for siblings of handicapped children, although it does seem
that the effects need not be negative, and indeed are often positive. Thus
some of the research in this area has indicated that siblings of children
with disabilities may develop a deeper understanding of people and of
handicaps, show more compassion, and have a better appreciation of
their own good health than their peers.

On the other hand, some siblings do seem to have problems in
emotional adjustment and well-being. Older sisters seem to be most at
risk in this respect, possibly as a result of being expected to take on more
of a child-rearing role in the family. Parents should therefore take pains
not to overburden their other children at home with responsibility.
Siblings have their *own* needs and, as far as possible, need time given to
them to foster their own development. Parents need to be particularly
alert to any hesitation their other children have in inviting friends home.
With younger children, it may be sensible for parents to talk with schoolfriends' parents to pave the way for having the friend round.

Telling your child with autism

More able children with autism may ask why they are different from
other children, and you may have to explain to them that they have a
handicap, what this means, and how it affects their lives. This is no easy
task. Broadly speaking the same approach we have advocated for siblings
is appropriate here. That is, parents need to be aware of the issues,
provide a suitable forum for discussion, share information at a pace
appropriate for their child, and pitch the content of what they say at a
level that can be understood. Understandably, children who recognize
their disabilities may become troubled by their handicap as its impact on
their lives becomes more evident. This is usually during adolescence and
early adult life, when the problems in establishing friendships persist

despite wishes to the contrary. Marked unhappiness may develop as a consequence. If this does emerge, parents should seek professional advice for their son or daughter.

Talking about the problems to friends and relatives

In addition to telling your other children, you will also have to let your parents and families know about your child with autism. It is as well to bear in mind that the news may be as distressing for grandparents as for you, although they may feel uneasy about sharing this with you. One particular area that some families feel sensitive about and which can cause difficulty concerns discussion about the possible hereditary factors involved in autism. It is important in this respect for families to be aware of the relevant information (discussed later in this book) while not getting caught up in unhelpful recriminations like 'it's not on our side of the family', etc. The issues are complex, and other close relatives planning a family may find it helpful to seek the advice of an expert in genetic counselling.

Much the same advice about talking to relatives also holds when dealing with friends and acquaintances—giving open and straightforward information about your child's handicap is the most effective way of preventing problems that emerge through ignorance or prejudice. This is often easier said than done. It can sometimes be quite challenging to think of ways of answering the critical looks or comments that you may get when your child behaves strangely in public. For advice on how to tackle these sorts of problems the best experts are usually other parents of children with autism.

Indeed, because of this, it is always recommended that parents should join the National Autistic Society or a similar parents' organization. In the UK, the National Autistic Society has a telephone help-line that can provide families with advice during the working week. Joining an organization such as the National or Local Autistic Society can also lead to discovering lots of practical tips, such as which hotels have an understanding and progressive policy towards people with disabilities—making holidays that much easier, or advice on what benefits one is entitled to. It can also lead to making contact with other parents in the same situation; and the discovery of how other people are coping can leave parents feeling less isolated or overwhelmed by the problems. Some parents even begin to feel that, with others, they can work to make the world a better place not only for their child, but for all children with autism.

4.

What causes autism?

The more difficult his behavior became, the more convinced I was that he was just doing it to spite me—to shut me out, to break my will, to win. I desperately wanted him to share in my world, but try as I might, everything was always on his terms. It was hard to believe that it might be a disease that was making him like this. I became embarrassed and afraid of taking him anywhere, believing that others would assume I was the cause of his strange behaviour. How could I convince them that it wasn't me, it was his brain? After all, he looked so normal.

In the last two chapters we reviewed the way in which a diagnosis is made, and the consequences of receiving the diagnosis. To recap, the diagnosis is made on the basis of three types of behaviour being present: abnormal social behaviour, abnormal communicative behaviour, and the presence of repetitive, unimaginative activities, all being evident in the first few years of life. In this chapter we summarize what is known about the cause or causes of autism that produce these abnormalities of behaviour. At the outset it is important to stress that no clear-cut answer exists on the question of cause; but what is known is discussed below.

The psychogenic theory of autism

It used to be thought that poor parenting caused autism—indeed, during the 1960s Bruno Bettelheim, a psychoanalyst and the author of a book on autism called *The empty fortress: infantile autism and the birth of the self* (Free Press, New York, 1967) advocated the practice of removing children from their parents as a means of treatment. Such a view is often referred to as the *psychogenic* theory of autism, and parents will be relieved to hear that it is entirely unsupported by any evidence.

In contrast, the *biological* theory of autism continues to be supported by growing evidence, year by year. The biological theory holds that in autism there are one or several abnormalities in the brain, and that these are caused by one or several biological factors (such as genes, complications during pregnancy or birth, or viral infections).

The biological theory of autism

There are several clues which lead to the conclusion that some biological abnormality is at the root of autism (summarized in Table 4.1). The most important of these is that autism is often accompanied by neurological symptoms, mental handicap, and certain medical conditions (such as epilepsy). In addition, the fact that autism is found with roughly equal frequency in different cultures suggests that social influences as a cause of the condition are unlikely.

Table 4.1: Some clues for the biological theory of autism

- *Features of the syndrome*
  —More often found in males
  —Roughly equally common in all areas and cultures

- *Associated factors*
  —Mental handicap
  —Epilepsy
  —Neurological symptoms
  —Minor congenital anomalies (birth defects)
  —Difficulties in pregnancy and labour

- *Links with other conditions*
  —Chromosomal/genetic conditions
  —Metabolic conditions
  —Viral infections
  —Congenital anomaly syndromes

It is difficult to grasp the plausibility of the biological theory when faced with the apparent contradiction that in many children there may be no apparent medical condition that has caused the autism, and no mental handicap or epilepsy. However, when *groups* of children with autism are studied, various medical conditions are found in association with autism more often than one would expect. The implication then is that in *all* cases some biological cause is likely to lie behind the autism, although currently this is only identifiable in a minority of cases.

In what follows, it is worth keeping in mind the point that a number of different factors can damage the brain, and that when any of these damage critical parts of the brain, the three key abnormal behaviours that characterize autism may be produced. The different factors that may damage the brain are discussed below.

Medical conditions which may cause autism

When autism occurs with a medical condition that can damage the nervous system, this is assumed to be the cause of the child's autism. The medical conditions that have been identified in some children with autism are listed in Table 4.2.

Table 4.2: Medical conditions found in autism (see Glossary for more details)

- *Genetic conditions*
  - —Fragile X syndrome
  - —Phenylketonuria
  - —Tuberous sclerosis
  - —Neurofibromatosis
  - —Other chromosomal anomalies

- *Viral infections*
  - —Congenital rubella
  - —Congenital cytomegalovirus
  - —Herpes encephalitis

- *Metabolic conditions*
  - —Abnormalities of purine synthesis
  - —Abnormalities of carbohydrate metabolism

- *Congenital anomaly syndromes*
  - —Cornelia de Lange syndrome
  - —Noonan syndrome
  - —Coffin Siris syndrome
  - —William's syndrome
  - —Biedl–Bardet syndrome
  - —Moebius' syndrome
  - —Leber's amaurosis

The list contains some conditions which are *genetic* (such as *tuberous sclerosis*), some which are *biochemical* (such as *phenylketonuria*), and some which are viral *infections* of the brain (such as the *rubella virus*). There are also a number of syndromes, termed *congenital anomaly syndromes*, that are sometimes seen in children with autism. This simply means that from birth there are identifiable physical abnormalities (for example, an unusually large head, or an abnormal position and formation of the ears).

All the medical conditions found in children with autism, though diverse, share the feature of being associated with brain damage or malfunction. However, it is worth stressing again that not everyone with autism has had these particular medical conditions, and indeed not everyone with these conditions develops autism. If your child does have one of these medical conditions, you should discuss in detail with your doctor how this may affect his or her future. Let us now look at each of these medical conditions in turn:

Genetic causes of autism

Does autism run in families?
About 2 or 3 per cent of brothers and sisters also develop autism. This rate is considerably higher than what would be expected from chance alone, and indicates that autism does indeed run in families. By itself, this finding does not give any clue to the cause of this family pattern; but the proof that genetic factors are involved comes from studies of twins.

Autism in twins
Identical twins (or 'monozygotic' twins) come from the same fertilized egg, and are therefore genetically identical. In contrast, non-identical (or 'dizygotic') twins develop from two separately fertilized eggs, and are therefore, in genetic terms, the same as any other brother or sister (that is, they share only half their brother's or sister's genes). In twin studies, scientists look at identical and non-identical twins in whom at least one has a disability. This type of study has been done for autism. The rate of both twins having autism in identical twins is indeed significantly higher than the rate in non-identical pairs. This is evidence that some genetic cause exists for autism. However, even in identical twins the chance of *both* twins having autism if one of them has it is not 100 per cent.

Some studies have checked for more general psychological difficulties in the twin who does not develop autism (such as language problems, mental handicap, or reading difficulties), and these studies have found that such difficulties occur quite often. This suggests that what is inherited may not simply be autism, but rather a range of psychological difficulties. About 10–15 per cent of the brothers and sisters of children with autism also have learning problems of this type. Parents may naturally be concerned by these findings, and watch anxiously for any signs of difficulty in the other children in the family. These worries should be discussed with the specialist. But it should be remembered that most brothers and sisters of children with autism develop normally.

Genetic conditions that can produce autism

There are a number of rare genetic conditions that can sometimes lead to autism. These are:

- *Phenylketonuria*

Phenylketonuria (or PKU) is an inherited condition involving an inability of the body to break down the naturally occurring chemical phenylalanine. As a consequence there is a build-up of related toxins in the body, and these in turn may damage the brain. The toxins are excreted in the urine. This problem is nowadays treated by putting babies with the abnormal gene on a special diet. Before the discovery of this treatment, children not only became brain-damaged but on occasions also developed autism. In the UK and in many other countries newborn children are tested in the first week of life to identify PKU, using a 'heel prick' blood test. If PKU is identified, treatment starts immediately. Fortunately, therefore, autism due to PKU is now very rare.

- *Neurofibromatosis (von Recklinghausen's disease)*

This genetic condition affects the nerves and skin, and mental handicap due to brain damage may also occur. The condition is often first recognized because there are a number of large brown spots (called *café-au-lait* spots) on the trunk of the body or on the limbs. Occasionally (but this is rare) children with neurofibromatosis also develop autism; but why this should be so is not known.

- *Tuberous sclerosis*

There are some studies indicating that autism is quite common in children who have the genetic condition tuberous sclerosis. However, because tuberous sclerosis is itself so rare, it is still an uncommon cause of autism. The features of tuberous sclerosis may include unusual skin pigmentation, a particular facial rash, and, most tragically, the growth of tumours in the brain, although not all of these features need be present.

Tuberous sclerosis may also give rise to a special form of epilepsy known as infantile spasms. This type of epilepsy has also been proposed as a cause of autism, so it is possible that the link between autism and tuberous sclerosis merely reflects the common association with infantile spasms. More recent evidence, however, questions whether this is the case, and suggests that it may be some other characteristic of tuberous sclerosis (possibly the location of tumours in the brain) that leads to the development of autism. Information about tuberous sclerosis is available from the Tuberous Sclerosis Association, a parents' and professionals' resource organization.

● *Fragile X syndrome*
Children with the fragile X syndrome usually develop mental handicap, and often have an unusual facial appearance (large protruding ears, a long nose, and a high forehead). The syndrome is called 'fragile X' because people with this condition have an abnormal gap on their X chromosome. Fragile X only occurs in a small proportion of children with autism (under 10 per cent); but this percentage nevertheless makes it the most common cause of autism yet identified.

● *Other conditions*
Moebius syndrome (a birth defect affecting the nerves controlling the eye and face muscles), and a number of other congenital anomaly syndromes (disorders characterized by particular contellations of defects that are present from birth) may produce autism (see Table 4.2).

If your child has any of these rare conditions, it will require specialist advice, in addition to the help your child may be receiving for autism. This should be discussed with your doctor.

To summarize the genetic evidence: a range of genetic conditions can cause autism, but these do not account for all cases of autism.

Difficulties in pregnancy and birth as possible causes of autism

Pregnancy and birth problems are more common in children with autism than one would otherwise expect. For example, the following 'risk' factors have been reported in association with autism:

- mothers above 35 years old at the time of the child's birth;
- birth order (first or fourth or later-born children may carry a slightly higher risk);
- medication during pregnancy;
- meconium (the first stools of the infant) was present in the amniotic fluid ('the waters') during the labour;
- bleeding between the fourth and eighth month of pregnancy; and
- a 'rhesus incompatibility' between the mother's and the child's blood groups.

The identification of these factors suggests that the difficulties in pregnancy or delivery may cause brain damage in the infant. However, it is important to remember that these factors are only evident in a minority of children with autism, and of course these factors also occur in the histories of many children who subsequently develop perfectly normally. So, *by themselves* they may not cause autism, but they may be *part* of the cause in some children. Just to complicate matters further, it is also the case that complications in pregnancy and delivery may be the *result* of the child's condition, rather than its cause. In such cases, the *original* cause of the child's autism may be genetic.

To summarize the pregnancy and birth evidence: a range of birth and pregnancy complications are associated with autism, but these factors alone are probably not sufficient to cause the condition. Rather, they may operate in combination with genetic or other factors, or merely indicate the presence of abnormalities already existing in the baby.

Infections as a cause of autism

As well as genetic and birth or pregnancy factors, infections that damage the brain during pregnancy or childhood are also associated with autism. It is assumed in these cases that the infections are causal, although, as with the birth complications, this need not be so. As yet the evidence is unclear in this respect. The infections that have been reported in association with autism are:

- *Rubella*
The rubella (or German measles) virus, particularly if contracted in the first three months of pregnancy, can damage the unborn baby's brain

and result in mental handicap, deafness, and blindness, as well as autism. With current vaccination programmes against rubella this is thankfully no longer a common problem.

● *Cytomegalovirus (CMV)*
The CMV virus can also result in mental handicap and, more rarely, autism. However, many newborn children who have been exposed to CMV have no apparent problems, so other factors must also operate to cause the difficulties in these cases.

● *Herpes encephalitis*
The herpes virus sometimes infects an infant's brain, and can lead to a brain inflammation known as encephalitis. Occasionally, children who develop herpes encephalitis are said to display an autistic-like condition. However, as with the other viral infections mentioned above, it should be remembered that many children who suffer a brain infection do not develop autism, and that the majority of children with autism had no apparent history of brain infection. This means that, for many children with autism, the cause of their problems still remains to be found.

To summarize the viral evidence: viruses that effect the brain in young infants or in the fetus may contribute to the cause of autism.

The idea of a 'final common pathway'

It is clear, then, that several medical conditions may predispose a child to developing autism. Even so, in the majority of children a medical condition cannot be found. To account for this puzzle, one model that has been proposed is known as the *final common pathway*, illustrated in Fig. 1. In this model, various causes of autism (some of which have yet to be discovered) all share the characteristic of damaging regions of the brain that are responsible for the development of normal communication, social functioning, and play.

It may be that mental handicap is associated with autism because the damage from these various medical causes also disrupts those systems in the brain that are necessary for intellectual development. Precisely which part of the brain is responsible for autism, or where this system is, is a problem scientists are tackling right now, in many different centres

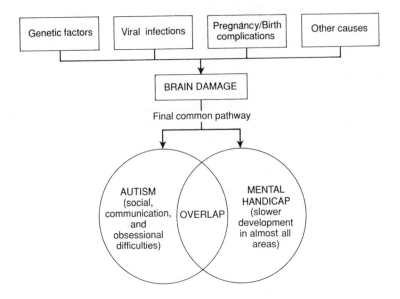

Fig. 1   The final common pathway to autism (one of several possible models).

around the world. But, despite our not having a definitive answer yet, the evidence that brain abnormalities exist in autism is no longer seriously doubted.

5.

The brain

The hardest thing for me to accept is that an abnormality of the brain produced the symptoms of autism. They haven't found anything wrong with John's brain. My doctor told me that I just have to accept it, because in other children with autism they have found brain damage. Sometimes I just look at him and think this is all wrong: surely he's got a normal brain and it's just a matter of time before he comes back to me?

The assumption is that in all children with autism there is some (possibly very subtle) brain damage. Where none can be found, it is assumed that this is because our tools for examining the brain are still too crude. Such brain damage, either observed or assumed, is held to cause the autism, as was made clear in the previous chapter. Parents often wonder if there really is any brain damage in their child, since he or she *looks* so normal. As we shall see, the brain-damage view is widely held simply because in many cases brain abnormalities *are* found. Here is the evidence.

Post-mortem studies

These studies have revealed abnormalities in different regions of the brain in different children and adults with autism. Abnormalities have been found in many areas, but usually either in the *frontal lobes* (responsible for planning and control, among other things), or in the *limbic system* (responsible for emotional regulation, among other things), or in the *brain stem* and *fourth ventricle*, or in the *cerebellum* (responsible for motor co-ordination, among other things). Figures 2, 3, and 4 show these areas of the brain. No single abnormality has been found in all of these post-mortem brain studies, and it is still uncertain which abnormalities are due specifically to autism, rather than to the accompanying mental handicap, or (in some cases) epilepsy.

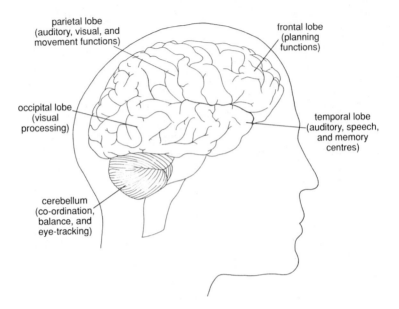

Fig. 2 The right cerebral hemisphere.

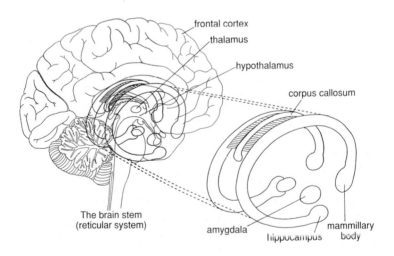

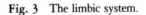

Fig. 3 The limbic system.

Brain scans

Various techniques have been developed for obtaining pictures of the brain. These include CAT (*Computed Axial Tomography*) scans, MRI (*Magnetic Resonance Imaging* scans, PET (*Positron Emission Tomography*) scans, and SPET (*Single Photon Emission Tomography*) scans. All of these types of scans have been used in autism research. The findings are bewilderingly wide-ranging, with abnormalities in different children being found in many different parts of the brain. As with the post-mortem examinations, there is no clear evidence of a specific abnormality occurring in autism only, and not in other conditions.

In one recent Californian study using the MRI scanner, cerebellar abnormalities were found in many (but not all) the children and adults with autism scanned. Similar cerebellar abnormalities have also been reported in people who have *fragile X syndrome*. Since this disorder is sometimes associated with autism, the finding of similar problems in the two conditions may be very important. The cerebellar abnormalities

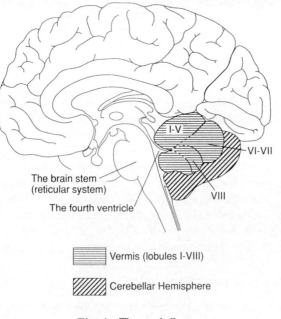

Fig. 4   The cerebellum.

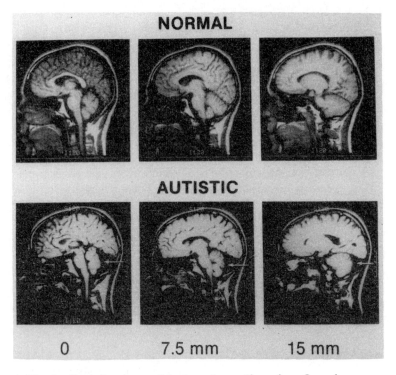

Fig. 5 Cerebellar abnormalities in autism: evidence from Courschesne.

from the scans of some people with autism are most evident in the part
of the cerebellum known as *vermal lobules VI-VIII* (shown in Figs 4
and 5). As can be seen, the lobules seem to be smaller in these cases of
autism. It has recently been proposed that these lobules may play a role
in the control of attention, among other things, though this claim
remains controversial. Several other research centres have failed to
identify cerebellar abnormalities of this type in the people they have
scanned, so the results of this study are currently unconfirmed by rep-
lication by other research groups. This is one of the crucial steps that
needs to be taken before results can be generally accepted.

Electrical activity of the brain

There are a number of methods for studying the way the nervous system
operates. Most of these methods involve measuring the electrical signals

emitted by the brain and its nerves while they are functioning. The best known means of measuring brain electrical activity involves the EEG (*electroencephalogram*). Using the EEG (which simply involves attaching wires to the scalp), researchers have examined electrical activity in the brain in people with autism. As with the postmortem and scanning investigations, no clear cut abnormality has been found. The EEG is also used in assessing epilepsy. A minority of people with autism do suffer from epilepsy, and this is discussed in more detail in Chapter 10.

When the brain perceives a light or a noise, it responds with a specific burst of electrical activity which can then be measured. This response is called an *event-related potential*. Measurement of these event related potentials in children with autism has revealed abnormalities in the brain's processing of novel sounds. This finding may be related to the observation that some children with autism occasionally cover their ears as if wishing to block out sounds or change their quality, and it may reflect unusual functioning of the auditory centres of the brain. This link remains to be tested further.

Brain chemistry

The only brain chemical that has clearly been found in abnormal levels in autism is *serotonin*. This is a neurotransmitter (i.e. a chemical responsible for transmitting signals in nerve cells). It has been discovered that between 30 per cent and 50 per cent of children with autism have abnormally high levels of serotonin in the blood. Exactly why the levels are high is not known. In children with mental handicap alone, serotonin may also be elevated.

The frontal lobe theory of autism

Recently, a new theory of autism has been proposed which suggests that many of the psychological features of autism can be accounted for by postulating abnormalities in the frontal lobes of the brain, since patients who acquire brain damage in the frontal lobe often show similar psychological deficits. This theory is currently generating new research. We shall return to this theory in the next chapter.

Does every child with autism need a brain scan?

At present, brain scans of children with autism are not carried out routinely, but only if the specialist feels a scan is needed, either for research purposes, or in cases where this may be important in the care of the child (for example, when there is epilepsy). In such circumstances the reasons for a scan and the details of the procedure are explained to the parents. If parents have concerns about this, it is worth discussing them with the doctor. In fact, the procedure is very similar to a standard X-ray. Moreover, the scan can often be done without any need for sedation, although for a very anxious person a mild sedative can be helpful. Very occasionally, in very restless and disturbed children, it may be best for the child to have an anaesthetic.

In summary, using a variety of different procedures, many children with autism have been found to exhibit features that suggest their brain development is abnormal. Whilst no specific abnormality has been found to underlie all cases of autism, there are many new leads that have emerged.

6.

Psychological problems

Everyone told me not to worry, since John was so bright. After all, he was a wizard at jigsaw puzzles, and he could sing all the words to the songs on our records. But I wasn't reassured by these things. I still knew he was not developing as he should. He said bizarre things, and sometimes used words that no one else understood. He talked to strangers but often ignored the people he knew best! And all those endless drawings of vacuum cleaners that he produced or cut out of catalogues and made us stick up on his bedroom wall. Surely that was not normal?

In this chapter we go on to describe how the brain abnormalities thought to underlie autism may produce anomalies in psychological functioning. These two levels of description, the brain and the mind, are separated into two chapters for convenience, though of course ultimately they are inseparable. As we mentioned in Chapter 2, the three key psychological problems in children with autism are in the development of social relationships, of language, and of the imagination. These need a closer look in order to try to understand them.

Social behaviour

An inability to relate socially to other people is the most important alarm signal when looking for autism. Leo Kanner, who first described autism (in 1943), gave what is perhaps still the clearest account of the social difficulties in these children. This indicates that there is no *single* social abnormality in autism, but rather there are a range of them. Extracts from the descriptions produced by Kanner (with his colleague Leon Eisenberg) are listed here:

- *unresponsiveness to people*
e.g.: 'He seems almost to draw into his shell and live within himself.'

- *lack of attention to people*
e.g.: 'When taken into a room, he completely disregarded the people and instantly went for objects.'

- *treating parts of people as detached objects*

e.g.: 'When a hand was held out to him so that he could not possibly ignore it, he played with it briefly as if it were a detached object.'

- *lack of eye-contact*

e.g.: 'He did not respond to being called, and did not look at his mother when she spoke to him.'

- *treating people as if they were inanimate objects*

e.g.: 'He never looked up at people's faces. When he had any dealings with persons at all, he treated them, or rather parts of them, as if they were objects. He would use a hand to lead him. He would, in playing, butt his head against his mother as at other times he did against a pillow. He allowed his boarding mother's hand to dress him, paying not the slightest attention to her.'

- *lack of behaviour appropriate to cultural norms*

e.g.: 'At two years old, she was sent to a nursery school, where she independently went her way, not doing what the others did. She, for instance, drank the water and ate the plant when they were being taught to handle flowers.'

- *attention to the non-social aspects of people*

e.g.: 'At the Child Study Home she soon learned the names of all the children, knew the colour of their eyes, the bed in which each slept, and many other details about them, but never entered into any relationship with them.'

- *lack of awareness of the feelings of others*

e.g.: '. . . on a crowded beach he would walk straight toward his goal irrespective of whether this involved walking over newspapers, hands, feet, or torsos, much to the discomfiture of their owners. His mother was careful to point out that he did not intentionally deviate from his course in order to walk on others, but neither did he make the slightest attempt to avoid them. It was as if he did not distinguish people from things, or at least did not concern himself about the distinction.'

- *lack of 'savoir-faire'*

e.g.: 'Even the relatively "successful" children exhibited a lack of social perceptiveness. This can be best illustrated by the following incident involving one of our patients who had made considerable progress. Attending a football rally of his junior college and called upon to speak, he shocked the assembly by stating that the team was likely to lose—a prediction that was correct but unthinkable in the setting. The ensuing round of booing dismayed this young man, who was totally unable to comprehend why the truth should be unwelcome.'

All these descriptions highlight the lack of normal social interest and social understanding. They also make it clear that not all children with autism are 'in a world of their own'. Some, like John whom we described in Chapter 1, do spontaneously approach other people, but sometimes only to carry out some repetitive, idiosyncratic preoccupation, such as touching another person's clothes or hair, or asking someone a limited set of questions. One of the questions that John often asked people in shops was 'What colour is your front door?'; but he never asked about people's feelings or thoughts.

The classic picture of 'aloneness' (see Fig. 6) is seen most often in younger children with autism—those of less than five years old. As they

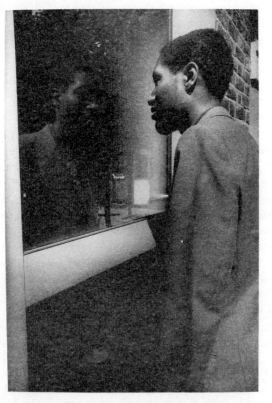

Fig. 6 Classical social 'aloneness' in autism.

get older they often become more outgoing. One important point to take from Kanner's descriptions is that if people with autism become more outgoing socially, this does not necessarily mean that their social behaviour has become 'normal'.

Response to other people

Children with autism are not completely unresponsive to others. For example, they tend to respond if others take the initiative in making social contact with them, especially if that contact is simple and clear. Nevertheless, they are unresponsive in other ways. For example, children with autism often show no *joint attention*. This means that, unlike other children, they don't attempt to catch another person's eye to show them toys, or share or point to things. They don't attempt to find out if the things that they are interested in are also of interest to other people, or to see if someone is trying to show them something of interest. This is part of what makes living with a child with autism such hard work. Parents try to share things with their child, but rarely does this happen the other way around. If the child does this at all, it is often in a very repetitive way.

Eye-contact

It is often claimed that children with autism avoid eye-contact with others. However, studies suggest that children with autism simply look for shorter periods at everything, and not less at the eyes in particular. This may give other people the impression that they are 'avoiding' eye-contact, whereas in reality it may not be so deliberate. Nevertheless, there is something odd about their use of eye-contact. They do not seem to understand how to use eye-contact to communicate 'without words', or to 'read' other people's faces. This means that often children with autism simply miss the exchange of glances that to the rest of us convey so much. They also don't seem to look at people's eyes and faces to read people's *intentions*, unlike even quite young normal children.

Emotions and relationships

Many young children with autism do have relationships with their parents, in that they appear to be emotionally 'attached' to their parents. Some children also showed the 'social smile' at the normal age of six weeks old, and continue to smile in an affectionate way; but this does not mean that their relationships are normal. For example, when John's favourite teacher left the school permanently, he repeatedly asked why she had left and even said that he missed her and wished she would come back. However, his reaction might have been simply due to the change in routine, rather than being a sign of a real relationship. Similarly, when John talks of having a 'friend', this often turns out to be just someone he has met once or twice, rather than meaning any deeper relationship.

The emotions children with autism show within relationships can also be quite unexpected. For example, most show the simple emotions of anger, fear, joy, and sadness, but they sometimes do so in situations when normal people would not show these. Lucy often laughs for no apparent reason; but neither she nor John show the more sophisticated emotions of pride, shame, or embarrassment. Alice, a teenage girl with autism we met recently, walked into the living room of her parents' home, completely naked, while we were talking to her parents. She did not show any signs of embarrassment, but simply approached us and said 'Do you watch weather forecasts on television?'

Understanding other people's thoughts

Children with autism have severe problems in taking other people's thoughts into account. They can understand what other people *see* (for example, if you ask people with autism 'What am I looking at?', they can answer correctly) but they show immense difficulty in the ability to appreciate other people's *thoughts*. This difficulty shows up on a test using a short puppet story (drawn in Fig. 7). In this story, Sally puts her toy in her basket and then goes out, but then while she is away, Anne moves it to her box. When children with autism are asked where, on her return, Sally thinks her toy is, they tend to answer that Sally thinks it is in Anne's box (where it *really* is), rather than the basket, where Sally *thinks* it is. They do not seem to appreciate that since Sally did not see her toy being moved into the box, she can't *know* it is there. They fail to take into account what another person thinks.

Because children with autism are unable to think about other people's thoughts, people's actions can appear very confusing to them, since the reasons people do things are often because they *think or believe* certain things. This may be one part of the explanation for the social abnormalities in autism. It may also explain their odd use of language, in that they frequently don't stop to check what their listener thinks or if their listener understands what they are saying.

The ability to think about other people's thoughts normally develops very early in life. Normal children and adults use this ability all the time in their dealings with the social world and in their understanding of

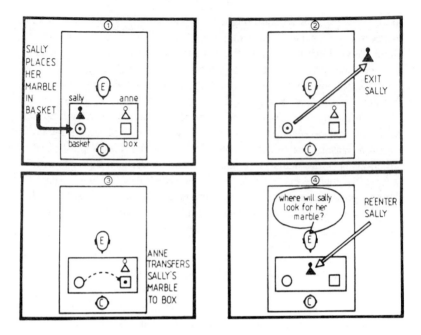

Fig. 7 The Sally-Anne test of a 'theory of mind'.

stories about people's lives. Take some of the first stories we tell young children. In *Snow White* the plot hinges on the fact that Snow White *thinks* she's being given a tasty apple—she doesn't *know* it really contains poison, and that the woman giving her the apple is really her wicked step-mother! (see Fig. 8).

Children with autism often fail to understand the deception involved in both fiction and real social life, precisely because they are unaware of what people are thinking, or of what people are trying to make others think. Psychologists refer to this as a failure to develop a concept (or a theory) of mind. Even more graphically, autism has been described as *mindblindness*, in an attempt to convey how out of touch children with autism are with what goes on in other people's minds. Whether this abnormality is open to treatment is not yet known. However, it leaves children with autism wide open to potential exploitation, simply because they cannot understand the concept of deception. This vulnerability can create special management problems in everyday life. Just as they have trouble understanding people's thoughts, so they also have difficulties in

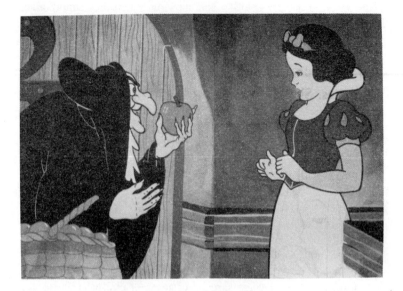

Fig. 8 The deception of Snow White.

recognizing and understanding emotions, beyond a very basic level. Certainly, understanding more complex emotions, such as embarrassment or surprise, may be completely beyond all but the most able individuals with autism.

Language

Apart from the social difficulties discussed above, language difficulties constitute another major set of problems. A range of communication difficulties exist, on many levels.

Preverbal communication

Normal children use many different types of communicative behaviour by the end of their first year. One set of behaviours briefly mentioned earlier are *joint-attention behaviours*. These include *pointing* in order to request objects, or to comment to another person about some object or event, and *showing and giving* objects to other people in order to communicate their interest in the object, or their desire for it. Children with autism rarely show any pointing and showing. Often they simply grab the object, ignoring the adult or other child who is holding it.

Non-verbal communication

Normal children and adults use gestures to accompany speech or to express emotions, embellishing these with the appropriate eye-contact and facial expressions. This non-verbal communication is also abnormal in autism, facial expression often not matching intonation, or gesture being out of step with speech. As we shall see, speech itself is abnormal too.

Abnormalities in speech

Many children with autism never develop any useful speech at all—that is, they never produce sounds that are recognizable as words. These children (such as Lucy, described in Chapter 1) are therefore described as functionally mute. For such children, communication problems are paramount, and even attempts at using non-speech systems (such as sign-language) may be relatively limited in success. In those children with autism who do develop speech, a variety of unusual features are sometimes (but not always) seen. These include:

● *echolalia*

These are words or phrases which are echoed either immediately after they are heard, or some time later. Many normal children go through a period when they echo speech, so it is important to determine if this echolalia is outside the normal range. A useful rule of thumb is that in normal children echoing stops by about the age of three. In autism echoing is often persistent beyond this point, and thus abnormal.

● *metaphorical language*

Whenever John, described in Chapter 2, wished to use the swing in the garden, he always said 'Go green riding.' In this example the 'metaphor' could only be understood if one knew John and the incident in which this phrase was first used. It should be noted that this is not a genuine metaphor in the sense that this term is used in linguistics.

● *neologisms*

Neologism literally means 'new word'. An example would be the word 'willip', which John created and used to mean a piece of fluff. Again, neologisms are also heard in normal children's language, but these do not usually persist in the face of other people's failing to understand them, unless it is in the context of a joke.

● *pronoun reversal*
(or difficulty with the use of pronouns). Children with autism may use
'you' when they mean 'I', or they may call themselves by their first
name. When his teacher asked 'Have you been swimming today?', John
often replied 'You been swimming today', meaning 'Yes, I've been
swimming.'

Language systems

When speech scientists study language, they divide it up into several
subsystems, and children with autism show abnormalities in each of
these.

One subsystem of language is *phonetics*, the system that produces
sound for speech. An abnormality in this system that has been found is
odd intonation. John's speech, for example, sounds mechanical and
monotonous. When this occurs, this may be part of a more general
failure to use language to communicate feelings and interest.

A second subsystem of language is the child's store of words, or
vocabulary. Acquisition of vocabulary in children with autism may
proceed at the normal rate, or it may be delayed. Many children with
autism who do speak eventually acquire large vocabularies, and may take
an obsessional interest in word-meanings. Other children with autism
may start speaking late. Failure to speak by the age of five years old may
be a sign that a poorer outcome can be expected. Nevertheless, some
children with autism do start to speak for the first time after the age
of five.

A third subsystem of language is *syntax*. Syntax refers to the rules of
grammar which allow us to combine words into meaningful phrases, and
to understand how word-order changes the meaning of phrases. Speech
in many children with autism contains the same syntax as is found in
normal children, and this is often acquired in the same sequence as it is
in normal children, even though there may be some delay in the acquisition process. The exception to this is with those parts of speech that have
shifting meanings—the *deixis* of speech. (Examples of *deixis* are
'here/there', 'now/then', and 'you/I'). Children with autism have enormous difficulties with these parts of speech.

Another subsystem of language is *semantics*. Semantics refers to the
rules describing the relationship between a word and the thing it describes—rules which allow us to use a word meaningfully. Children with
autism who can speak also use words to refer to things, but show characteristic problems with the meanings of more abstract or figurative

expressions. For example, words are often understood only on a very literal level. The phrase 'He cried his eyes out' provoked John to look for eyes on the floor. He also could not accept that two expressions (for example, 'door-handle' and 'door-knob') could refer to the same thing, or that two different objects could have the same name ('bank', for example, meaning both a place where you keep your money, and the land at the side of a river).

A final subsystem of language is *pragmatics*. Pragmatics refers to the rules of conversation that enable us to use language in ways that are appropriate to the social context and the listener. Children with autism often use language in ways that are inappropriate to the social context. One of the clearest examples of this is seen in echolalia, when the child repeats a word, a phrase, or even a whole section of conversation he or she has heard before, out of context. Another abnormality in pragmatics is evident in the difficulty in recognizing the *intention* behind someone's speech, that is, in inferring what the other person expects of one in a conversation. For example, if normal children are asked 'Do you know where Mummy is?', they do not simply reply 'Yes' (unless they are trying to be either funny or uncooperative). In contrast, children with autism may give a 'yes' answer to questions of this kind, not for reasons of wanting to be funny or difficult, but simply because they do not realize that the other person was *expecting* more or different information.

Language teaching to overcome these problems is a key focus in the education of children with autism, and we shall return to this in Chapter 8.

Repetitive, obsessional behaviour

So far we have described in detail the problems children with autism have in social and language development. The third and final area of difficulty that makes up the diagnosis is a lack of flexible imagination, coupled with obsessional behaviour. John, you may recall, took an obsessional interest in counting lampposts, collecting bottle-tops, and naming geometric shapes. This repetitive quality in the interests of children with autism makes their play very uncreative. So, for example, *pretend play*, normally seen from about 18 months onwards, in which the child creatively uses an object as if it were some other object (for example, using a cup as if it were a hat), is rarely seen in children with autism. If it is present at all, it is usually very limited. Its absence or limited appearance immediately alerts the professional to the possibility of autism.

Recently, psychological research has also uncovered severe difficulties in *planning skills* in children with autism, combined with the presence of a rigid, perseverative approach to problem solving. Such difficulties are sometimes referred to as *executive* problems and are thought to be due to abnormalities in the frontal lobes of the brain. It is quite possible that such psychological anomalies underlie the obsessional behaviour typically seen in autism.

Dealing with the child's obsessions can be the most difficult part of home life. Some ideas for overcoming obsessions are suggested in Appendix 3. It should be stressed that repetitive rituals, whilst a key feature of autism, are not always particularly marked in all children. Some have many preoccupations, evident in their play (for example, repeatedly lining things up around the house) or their school-work (for example, putting a little dot after each word when they write) or their interests (for example, listening to all the weather forecasts on the radio) or their eating habits (for example, insisting on only one brand of sausages, to be served on the same plate each time). Other children with autism have less marked obsessional behaviour.

The problems in social and communicative development, and in flexible thinking, are psychological; but ultimately they have their cause in abnormalities in the brain, as we pointed out in Chapter 5. Understanding the links between the psychological and the brain abnormalities is one of the most important areas of current research.

7.

Intelligence and special talents

Sometimes I wondered, as I stared at him drawing swiftly and confidently but with no regard for who saw the picture or whether it ultimately was thrown away, whether his autism was something that just went hand in hand with being a 'genius'. I was proud of his talent (although most other people soon lost interest in his drawings of canal locks). But what use, I thought, was such ability when he couldn't even play properly, or sympathize with others, or realize when people were taking the mickey out of him and pulling the wool over his eyes?

This chapter continues our summary of psychological abnormalities in autism from the last chapter, but focuses specifically on intelligence and special talents. This merits its own chapter because of the finding that intelligence is often unusual in autism, and that special abilities are more commonly associated with children with autism than with other conditions.

Intelligence

Intelligence is a difficult thing to define. However, we need not get bogged down in definitions here. Instead, for the present purposes, we can define intelligence as those abilities that are measured by IQ (or 'Intelligence Quotient') tests. When IQ is measured at different times over a person's life, it is found to be approximately the same, give or take about 15 points. For example, if a child is in the average IQ range (70–130) at the age of 8 years old, then he or she is also likely to be in this range of scores at any stage in the future. If a person's IQ is below the average range (i.e.: less than 70) he or she may have difficulties in learning, and require special education. In such cases, people are said to have a mental handicap.

The old view that children with autism cannot have their IQ tested is not supported by evidence, although it is true that some children with autism under the age of five years old are partially untestable because they cannot sit still for long enough to complete all the tests. Even with these children, some estimates of their abilities can be made on the basis of the few tests they do complete. In testing any person with autism, examiners need to be highly experienced to obtain meaningful results.

IQ test scores of children with autism provide a reasonably good way of predicting what their eventual educational and social outcome is going to be like. This is particularly important because, as was mentioned earlier, approximately two-thirds of children with autism score in the below-average range (less than 70). Their low IQ scores are not due to lack of motivation, because when given tests which are within their level of ability they often appear to be highly motivated. Neither are these results simply a consequence of language delay, since some children with autism perform poorly on verbal tests, but normally on non-verbal tests. We should remember that however well a child with autism does on an IQ test, these are tests (often) of logic and perception. They give no estimate of social understanding, which may be very poor even in a person of high IQ.

Islets of ability in autism

Children with autism often perform well in tests that involve visual–spatial ability, such as jigsaw puzzles. Sometimes, these are the only good skills a child has. When this occurs the skills are sometimes referred to as isolated *islets of intelligence*. Leo Kanner considered these to be characteristics of autism. By this he meant that they occur commonly in autism, although they are not present in all cases. Sometimes children with autism are even superior in their islet of ability to normal children of the same chronological age. The best-documented examples of islets of ability in autism are in drawing, music, and calendar calculation. Other skills which have also been described include rote-memory, finding shapes within patterns, and hyperlexia (precocious reading). These special skills are sometimes also called *savant abilities*, and these can also occur in conditions other than autism. For example, there are reports of individuals who have moderate mental handicap (with IQs often as low as 40–50), but who are talented in one area only. Many such individuals also have autism. This implies that, although independent, autism and savant abilities must be related in some way, though this link still is not well understood.

When a person with autism shows a markedly developed islet of ability, he or she may be referred to as an 'autistic savant'. This term was first coined by Bernard Rimland and was used to describe the character played by Dustin Hoffman in the film *Rain Man*. Some of the main islets of ability found in autism are described next.

Unusual drawing ability

One of the first carefully documented cases of a child with autism with extraordinary drawing ability was that of Nadia, a girl with hardly any language. Her drawings were remarkable for a number of reasons. For a start, they did not fit the stages of development seen in normal children. For example, she drew things in perspective at the age of three, whereas normal children tend not to achieve perspective in drawing until at least adolescence, and many of us never master it at all. Nadia's drawings were highly repetitive in theme, reflecting her obsessional interests, but each drawing showed different perspectives of the image she was looking at. For example, at the age of three she was obsessed with horses, and drew hundreds of horses over the next few years, from different angles, and with incredible vividness and accuracy (see Figs 9 and 10).

Many of her drawings are very literal: in a sense, they capture what the eye actually sees, in an almost photographic way. All the more

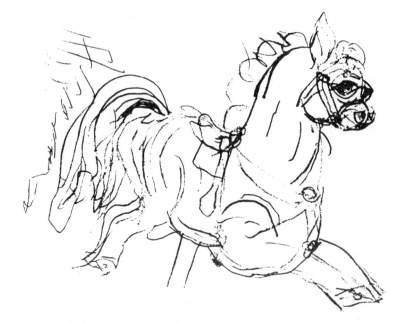

Fig. 9   Drawing by Nadia, aged 3½ years old.

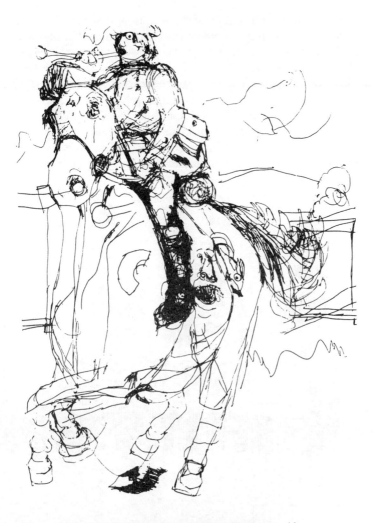

Fig. 10 Drawing by Nadia, aged 5 years old.

remarkable in Nadia's case was the fact that she did not sit and study real horses, but drew her pictures after seeing a horse in a story book. From this she generated endless numbers of images of what a horse should look like in any posture. Most mysteriously, as Nadia began to speak, around the age of 11, she gradually produced fewer drawings, and now produces only occasional sketches.

Other children with autism with remarkable drawing ability have since been reported, much of whose work shows similar features to that of Nadia. One boy who has recently had his work published is Stephen Wiltshire, whose obsessional theme is drawing buildings. Unlike Nadia, his drawings are derived from personal experience of these objects, and he has drawn many of the important buildings in New York, London, and other cities. His pictures of St Paul's Cathedral and The Eiffel Tower are shown in Figs 11 and 12. His drawings are all the more incredible when compared with the real buildings: details such as the style and size of windows of ornate buildings are recorded faithfully, and this is despite

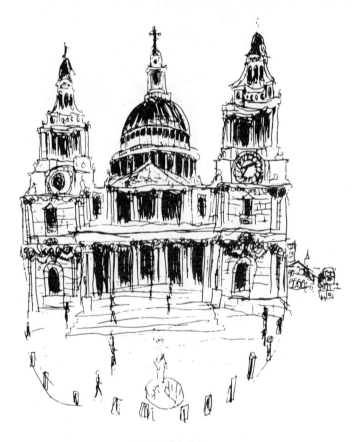

St Paul's Cathedral

Fig. 11   Drawing by Stephen Wiltshire.

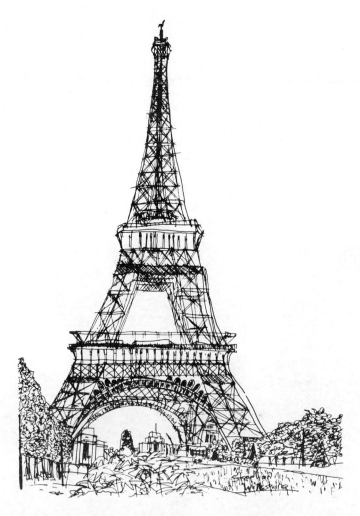

Eiffel Tower

Fig. 12 Drawing by Stephen Wiltshire.

Stephen only having viewed the original building once, for a few brief minutes, and often not beginning his drawing until he has returned to his home or school. It should however be noted that many children with autism show no unusual drawing talent.

Musical ability

Many children with autism love to listen to music, and sometimes can sing long passages very accurately. For example, Lucy (who we described in Chapter 1) could hum long passages from Tchaikovsky that she had heard her mother play on the piano. Some children with autism have special musical talents, such as the ability to play instruments they have never been taught, the ability to produce complex melodies accurately on such instruments after hearing the melody just once (see Fig. 13), and the ability to name any note they hear (perfect or absolute pitch). This is not just a case of remarkable 'parroting', because these children are also sensitive to the structure of music, recognizing its repeating themes and phrases, as well as being able to reproduce it in different keys. Again, like unusual drawing ability, this is quite rare.

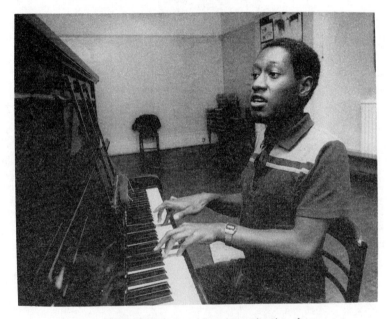

Fig. 13   Musical talent in autism, in a minority of cases.

Rote-memory and calculation skills

Rote-memory is often observed in children with autism: they seem to store lists of items in memory for prolonged periods in the exact form in which they were first experienced, again without changing them in any way. For example, John (in Chapter 1) often narrated the words of television advertisements, or lists of makes of cars. Another quite rare phenomenon which was once thought to be an example of rote memory is *calendar calculation*. This is the ability to say on which day of the week any date will fall. However, this cannot simply be an example of rote-memory, as there are many dates in the distant past or future for which calendars do not exist and which could not therefore have been memorized. Rather, children with autism who have this ability seem to have a knowledge of the rules governing calendars, and apply these rules automatically—that is, without knowing how they do it—and very rapidly. Indeed, they can sometimes be quicker at it than mathematicians who have consciously worked out the formulae. This phenomenon is also occasionally seen in another form, *mathematical calculation*, in which some children can mentally add, subtract, multiply, or divide large numbers, sometimes even faster than someone using a hand calculator.

Other islets of ability

There are many accounts of children with autism being able to do jigsaw puzzles not only at the appropriate age-level, but also at more advanced levels, and even picture-face down, as John was able to. This suggests that they do not need to rely on the picture in order to identify the position of the piece in hand, but can use other clues, such as its shape or feel. There are also many anecdotal reports of good constructional skills in young children with autism who, having dismantled record-players and other quite complex machines, can reassemble them.

Quite what causes some children with autism to be so talented is still not known. Practice may be part of the explanation, but some children show these skills even from a very young age (like Nadia), and without much practice. Rather, these areas of special ability (like the social and language difficulties described in the previous chapter) are likely to reflect an unusual organization of the brain in autism.

Should I encourage my child's special talent, if he or she has one?

If your child has a talent such as drawing or memory skills, by all means encourage it. Sometimes parents worry that by allowing their child to engage in their well-practised activity, this will block opportunities for development in other areas. There are no hard answers available here, but it seems reasonable both to develop the child's talents *and* provide opportunities for other experiences too.

8.

Education: what can be done?

I wanted a school where he could be himself, where he wouldn't be teased or bullied for being different, where they would understand him. But most of all I wanted a school where they would patiently work at getting through to him. If they could do it, I felt sure he could make huge strides and become more independent of us eventually. Our biggest worry was that if his education failed him, he would not be able to cope on his own when we were old, or after we were gone.

It used to be thought that children with autism were ineducable, as was mentioned in Chapter 1. In the past such attitudes resulted in children with autism being placed in the back wards of long-stay mental-handicap institutions, and their lack of progress was then taken as proof of their ineducability. When such assumptions were questioned in the case of children with mental handicap, and discovered to be wrong, their validity for autism was also challenged. Current evidence suggests that very few, if any, children are ineducable—whatever their intellectual level. The overriding principle is that education should be tailored to the individual, and educability is evident in the progress made, whatever its rate.

What kind of educational setting is best?

Highly structured teaching programmes have been claimed to produce the greatest gains. There are several reasons why this may be so. First, the social problems in autism are such that, if a teacher is not actively initiating interaction and being directive, a child with autism may simply drift away from social contact into a pursuit of repetitive patterns of behaviour. Such repetitive behaviours, by definition, allow very little learning of new information. Secondly, the highly structured approach starts from the assumption that every task should be broken down into simple and clear steps, with each goal clearly defined. Children with autism seem to take to such a methodical approach. Finally, highly structured teaching may work because children with autism seem to prefer predictability. They like the fact that, for example, on Wednesdays it is cooking in the morning and art in the afternoon, while on Thursdays it is maths in the morning and music in the afternoon. Sudden and apparently unexplained changes in the timetable can lead to tantrums or distress. Structure and predictability of course still need to leave room for flexibility and spontaneity. Indeed, flexibility may need to be specifically worked at so that children with autism do not end up totally unprepared for the 'real world'. Certainly, attempts to teach 'social skills' in an inflexible way can be self-defeating, as normal social behaviour is by definition inherently flexible.

Choosing the right school

In many countries, the National Autistic Society and local Autistic Societies run some schools. Many are also run by Local Educational Authorities. Within the National Autistic Society schools in the UK, the model school combines structured teaching, to facilitate learning, with creative approaches, to facilitate the development of communication and social interaction. These more creative approaches include music, art, and drama therapy (described later). Other schools, not run by the National Autistic Society, also use this sort of model. Parents can seek advice about the relative merits of different types of school for different types of children from the National Autistic Society, or equivalent organizations (see Appendix 1). Choosing the right school is essential: it needs to be a school that understands the nature of the child's problems, and is open-minded in its attempts to find out what works. At present there is no *single* method that is right for all children with autism; teachers must be experimental enough to adapt methods to the individual.

What is the most effective teacher–pupil ratio?

If children with autism are not given individual attention, they may revert to their own repetitive activities or solitary existence. Some children with autism are able to work individually without anyone sitting at their side, sometimes for long periods of time, although this ability may develop quite late in some children (around 8–10 years old), and may need to be specifically taught. To maintain their attention sufficiently for learning to occur, a ratio of at most 3 pupils to 1 teacher seems appropriate. The National Autistic Society schools in the UK

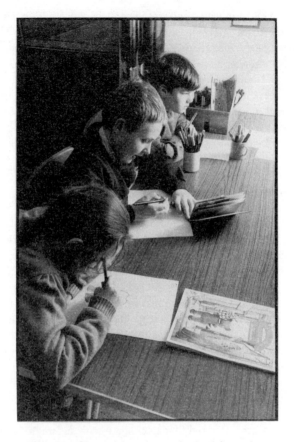

Fig. 14 Class-work in a special school for autism.

have aimed to meet this criterion by employing a teacher's assistant as well as a teacher for each class. Class sizes of 6 pupils are therefore standard in such schools. However, some smaller units for autism have sometimes found that a one-to-one teacher–pupil ratio is ideal, if resources allow.

What can be achieved?

Even with as little as two years of schooling, children with autism improve considerably in their educational development. Those who make educational progress also tend to have the best outcomes, although their IQ at five years old is also an important predictor of their eventual attainment. This last point means that for those children whose IQ is in the average or above-average range, academic attainments may also be normal. Some adults with autism have even gone through higher education and achieved college degrees. Temple Grandin, who holds a Ph.D. in Agricultural Science, and who has written a book about her personal experience of autism, is a rare example of such achievement.

Among children with autism of normal intelligence, school subjects that do not require extensive social or communicative skills are often preferred, probably because these subjects are learned more easily. Such subjects include maths, crafts, and music. Similarly, subjects in which children can use their often good memories for learning long lists of facts may be easier. By contrast, the study of literature, which involves the interpretation of a person's *meaning* and *intentions*, poses considerable difficulties for children with autism.

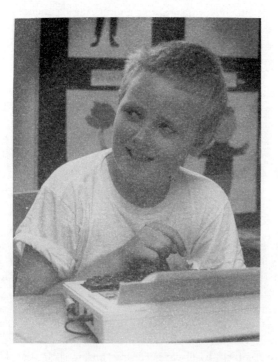

Fig. 15   The use of computers in the education of children with autism.

Since the majority of children with autism also have mental handicap, educational progress is often slower than normal. So by the time they leave school many may have only mastered basic skills, such as simple reading, writing, and understanding money and elementary arithmetic, sometimes acquired through the use of educational computer software (see Fig. 15). Many may also have succeeded to some extent in acquiring basic self-help skills, such as cooking, dressing, laundry, etc. These fundamental skills should not be taken for granted: they allow people with autism to participate to varying extents in our social world, and achieve some degree of independence.

Can communication be taught?

Sounds, words, and even sentences can be taught, to varying degrees, depending on the individual child's ability. Communication, though, is not just about producing sounds or grammatically correct sentences. Rather, it is about conveying *meaning* and sharing experiences through a social dialogue. In fact, producing grammatically correct sentences has very little to do with communication *per se*. So, as well as teaching words and sentences, it is important to encourage children to *use* phrases in a genuinely communicative way. Such training is really only in its infancy in many schools for autism, so we are not yet able to say how far such skills can be taught successfully. One exciting approach being developed in Sutherland House School, Nottingham, involves encouraging children with autism to use the *pointing* gesture and turn-taking, *before* expecting any other communicative development. Such creative approaches need evaluation.

Sign language

Sign language is sometimes used to help build communication in those children with speech difficulties. This is done either to improve expression (that is, if their speech is undeveloped and incoherent, a manual sign can often clarify which word they are using), or to improve their understanding of someone else's speech. In the latter case, it is argued that signs are more concrete and simpler to understand than spoken words. Signing can therefore make it that much easier for some children with autism to discover the meaning of language. However, sign language is best used as an aid to developing communication and speech. If it is taught as an end in itself, its obvious disadvantage is that the child is then restricted to communicating only with those who can understand signing. Speech should therefore be thought of as the communicative medium to teach, and signing as a stepping-stone towards this goal. However, not all children are able to develop speech, and for these children sign language may be vital. An example of sign language being taught at one British school for autism is shown in Fig. 16.

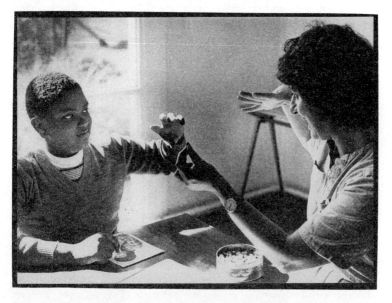

Fig. 16 The teaching of sign-language to children with autism who lack speech.

Statements of Educational Needs

In the UK and many other countries every child with autism requires a *statement* of his or her educational needs, prepared by an educational psychologist, in order to qualify for a special school, or for additional help (for example, a personal assistant-teacher) in a mainstream school. Following an evaluation, the educational psychologist and other professionals involved in the child's care compile a report for the local education authority. This sets the wheels in motion for getting access to the best school for that particular child. When the statementing procedure runs smoothly, it is a good way of ensuring the best for a child and keeping the child's needs under review. Parents are invited to comment on and contribute to the statement before it is finalized, so that parents should not feel inhibited in expressing their concerns and views.

It should be noted that parents sometimes experience difficulty at this stage, sometimes because the professionals have a different view of their child's educational needs, or more commonly, because the process is so protracted, with families having to fight bureaucracy at every stage. Another frequent disappointment is what has become known as 'resource-led statementing', meaning that the statement may be written only with a view to what is locally available rather than to what the child actually needs. Parents should therefore read the statement carefully to check that they agree with the details of the evaluation. We hope the system will become easier for parents to use. It is a source of frustration they can well do without.

Integration

Should children with autism be integrated into mainstream educational settings? Certainly one might think that placing children with autism together at school may simply compound the social problems of each child, since they may receive fewer opportunities to experience normal social interaction, compared to what happens in a mainstream school. On these grounds alone, it seems sensible to provide opportunities for children with autism to be among normal peers. This does not however mean that integration into mainstream schooling is necessarily better than education in separate units or schools for autism, since such specialist units often have expertise and resources that are hard to find in mainstream settings. Such resources include, for example, the teacher-pupil ratios discussed earlier. In addition, resources are often not available to prevent any stigmatization that might take place when a person with autism is placed in a mainstream school. At the present time, given the lack of resources, it may be better for children with autism to be educated in specialist units, while the child is given plenty of opportunities to mix with other children whenever feasible. Such integration is also likely to have additional benefits for the normal children they mix with, in terms of developing their awareness and understanding of the special needs of children with autism. Integration is a process that we need to facilitate at all possible opportunities.

9.

Other therapies

I wanted some good practical advice on how to deal with him when he threw things around, smeared food on the wall, and refused to wear clothes. In this, his head teacher was terrific. But I also wanted, prayed for, something that would get at the root of his autism, that would break through it or make it go away. Some things have worked a little, but we still keep hoping.

In the years since autism was first described, a range of different psychological treatments have been tried. While there have been no independently assessed demonstrations of an absolute cure, different kinds of psychological treatment have nevertheless had considerable beneficial effects. The clearest example is behaviour therapy, and this is described first.

Behaviour therapy

Behavioural programmes are designed by psychologists and psychiatrists working in consultation with parents, teachers, or care staff, and are essentially ways of shaping adaptive behaviours (such as toilet training) or decreasing maladaptive behaviours (such as spitting). As such, behaviour therapy can be of immense practical value. In behaviour therapy, the behaviour is analysed into its causes and consequences, and then a behavioural programme is implemented. The aim is to identify the factors that *reward* or encourage appropriate behaviours, as well as those that succeed in discouraging disruptive behaviours. Rewards need to be based on what each individual child values, and have to be given clearly and consistently. Modern behaviour therapy does not punish children for bad behaviour, as this is often ethically unjustifiable. Instead, it attempts to reduce such maladaptive behaviour by removing the factors that may be encouraging it, and replacing it with more positive skills.

Once a useful behaviour has begun to emerge, even in a primitive form (such as an attempt at a word by a mute child), additional techniques can then be used to increase and fine-tune the behaviour. Behaviour therapy can be useful in reducing such problems as self-injury (head-banging and self-mutilation), hyperactivity, aggression, and tantrums. It is also useful in increasing self-help skills (dressing, washing, etc.), occupational and, to some extent, educational skills. It has, for example, been used success-fully to increase speech quantity and quality. Unfortunately, despite these benefits, it has failed to affect significantly the social, com-municative, and imaginative abnormalities, because these do not solely depend on single behaviours (for example, eye-contact) that can be in-creased or decreased. Some applications of behaviour therapy to specific problems are listed in Appendix 3.

Social skills training

Social skills training is the name given to a broad range of techniques used to help teach children and adults with autism how to interact socially. Since each social situation is unique, and has its own set of 'rules', this is painstaking work for the teacher or therapist. But since it is precisely in this area that people with autism find most difficulty, it is an essential part of education and treatment. Examples of social skills training would be teaching adolescents with autism how to make phone calls, how to go shopping, or how to behave on the bus. In each case, it is not the physical aspects of the task (how to dial the phone-number, or how to count the money) which necessarily pose the difficulties, but the social conventions that surround these (how to start, maintain, and finish the phone-call, how to wait politely for one's turn in the supermarket queue, or how not to stare at people on the bus). The techniques to achieve this include role-play and video-feedback, as well as basic one-to-one teaching in real situations.

To some extent, these skills can be taught, although teachers often report difficulty in getting the child or adult with autism to *generalize* the skill to new situations, or to remember to use it. The final product, 'social behaviour', can also come across to other people as rather odd or stilted, simply because it has been acquired through systematic teaching rather than being learned 'naturally'. Finally, there are some important aspects of social skills which have proved very difficult to teach. These include 'empathy', or sensitivity to other people's thoughts and feelings.

The TEACCH Program

This programme, developed by Erich Schopler and his colleagues in North Carolina, has evolved over almost twenty years to cover most aspects of family services connected to autism. TEACCH stands for the Treatment and Education of Autistic and related Communication-handicapped CHildren. The treatment aspects include both language- and behaviour-focused intervention programmes, which are individually drawn up, as well as school and other agency consultation. This approach also works with parents, either by encouraging parent training and counselling, and/or facilitating parent support groups. This work has been evaluated in the US, and shows important benefits. These results are also mirrored to some degree in the *Home-Based Treatment Programme* developed by Patricia Howlin and Michael Rutter in London, which provides behaviour therapy and family support. The TEACCH programme also combines treatment with diagnostic and assessment methods.

Psychotherapy and autism

As a result of the *psychogenic* theory of autism (see Chapter 4) a number of psychiatrists and psychoanalysts advocated psychotherapy for parents of children with autism. Such psychotherapy was based on the principle that parents had to become better parents in order to allow their child to develop emotionally, and that psychotherapy was the route to allow such growth. However, neither the assumption about parenting causing autism, nor the claim that psychotherapy for parents leads to emotional development in their child, have been supported by any systematic evidence.

This is not to say that psychotherapy has no value for parents, or for people with autism themselves. The value of psychotherapy will of course depend on which particular kind of therapy is tried—there are a range of different kinds. Its main value in the context of autism is in providing supportive counselling, and working through difficult periods and the depression these may cause. To reiterate, psychotherapy based on the belief that parents cause their child's autism is nothing short of misguided; but, as in other situations, psychotherapy as an opportunity to deal with issues in a safe and impartial setting has distinct value. However, if psychotherapy is considered for individuals with autism themselves, it should be borne in mind that it is unlikely to be of use to those with insufficient language skills. The alternative non-verbal technique for children with autism is *play therapy*. This practice is valuable in helping children with autism to control anxiety and play more creatively, but it can be counterproductive if the therapist makes interpretations of the child's play that simply confuse the child.

Some specialist therapies

Music therapy

Music therapy is used in most special schools for autism, with good results. It has been found, for example, that with a skilled therapist, *turn-taking* can be developed, and this may be useful for social skills. Whether turn-taking in a music session generalizes to other situations has not been systematically investigated. But apart from using music to encourage communication in this way, music therapy has also been used to

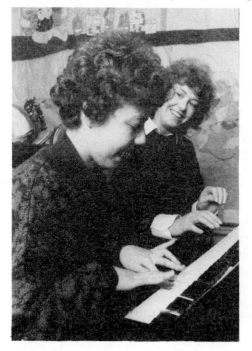

Figs 17 and 18   Music therapy in a special school for autism.

bring out what are often normal and even superior musical talents in children with autism.

Some children with autism demonstrate their musical skills without any special tuition—playing melodies they have heard just once, and with remarkable accuracy; but, as we have pointed out in Chapter 7, such 'savant' skills are seen in less than 5 per cent of children with autism. Others, with patient teaching, demonstrate their good 'feel' for rhythm and melody, and succeed in learning musical instruments. Perfect pitch—the ability to sing the exact note on which a melody starts without any external cue—seems to be present in a number of children with autism, and indeed may be more common in this group than in other clinical groups.

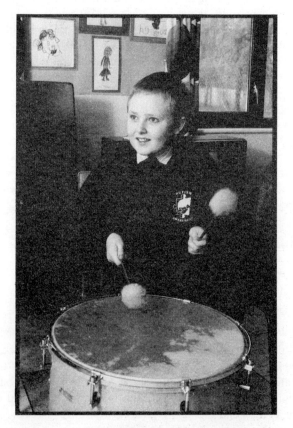

Fig. 18

Music therapy at the very least has a very calming effect on many children with autism, and it is reported that for some children singing is actually easier to understand than speech. Singing therefore lends itself to being used to facilitate communication in these cases. One excellent example of this is in *Music-Assisted Communication Therapy*, developed by Dawn Wimpory and Phil Christie in Nottingham.

Speech and language therapy

Speech and language therapy is the other specialist therapy that is found in many schools and units for autism, as well as being used during the preschool years, which has demonstrable benefits. Speech therapists (or the teachers they train) work on every level of language-development, from encouraging speech-like sounds in mute children with autism, to developing syntax in those with delayed language, to fine-tuning intonation and the 'pragmatic' aspects of speech in children with autism who speak in fully formed sentences. (As we explained in Chapter 6, 'pragmatics' refers to the social and communicative use of language.) They also attempt to develop comprehension. However, a realistic appraisal of speech and language therapy must conclude that, despite intensive individual treatment, spontaneous and appropriate conversational speech is difficult to encourage, even if the more 'technical' aspects of speech can be taught. But even these achievements, though limited, are nevertheless very valuable. Conversational skills may need to be encouraged in more natural settings, such as while playing at home. It may also be that speech therapy at an early stage in development would have more impact. This remains to be tested.

Some newer psychological treatments

In recent years, a number of psychological treatments have received considerable publicity in the media because of their claims of success with autism. Some of these are discussed next.

Holding therapy

Holding therapy was developed by Martha Welch in New York, and is practised in a number of centres around the world. In this therapy, parents are encouraged literally to hug their child for long periods, even if the child protests and tries to pull away. Using such forced holding techniques, the child eventually gives up resisting, and some parents report that the child begins to explore his or her parent's face and make better eye-contact. There are also some reports from parents that this leads to more normal social relationships and communication.

There can be little doubt that such intensive physical and social contact may produce changes, and some parents report that most of these changes are worthwhile. For example, some withdrawn children with autism become better able to tolerate being held. Others, who initially had little eye-contact, often develop the ability to maintain eye-contact for longer periods. There may be benefits for parents too: many report feeling physically closer to their child, and some report feeling that, for the first time, real affection is being shown by their child. However, one must also consider possible disadvantages. The main one seems to be that, as it appears to observers, many children with autism react to forced holding as if it is aversive—they fight to escape it. Naturally, if this process led to a cure, any possible suffering might be thought of as justifiable. However, there is as yet no evidence that holding therapy does cure autism, despite the claims by some practitioners. Certain behaviours may change, but this is a far cry from saying that the child's *understanding* of and communication with the social world has become normal. Furthermore, some children with autism show similar changes in behaviour but without going through holding therapy. This means that the changes may be due to factors other than holding *per se*. A scientific evaluation is needed to examine such factors further.

Daily Life Therapy

In Daily Life Therapy (as practised at the Higashi Schools in Japan and the United States), group activities are emphasized, and with the guidance of trained teachers, children with autism are put through intensive physical activities under a highly regimented schedule, without letting the child lapse into his or her autistic withdrawal. This method was developed by the late Dr Kiyo Kitahara, in Tokyo. Media reports have suggested that such 'regimes' lead to children with autism participating in more social activities, but to date there has been no scientific evaluation of this method. There can be dangers associated with vigorous exercise for children with autism, especially those who have epilepsy. For this reason, children with epilepsy are sometimes excluded from these schools. In their favour are the impressive arts programmes these schools offer, and the group activities which many children successfully learn to cope with.

Other therapies

In *Patterning Therapy* (described by Carl Delacato) children with autism are encouraged to use alternative sensory channels to overcome unusual sensitivities and to rejuvenate brain development. The *Walden Method*, named after its pioneer, the late Geoffrey Walden, aims to develop understanding and problem-solving skills in a gradual, step-wise approach through entirely non-verbal tasks, in which the child takes the lead. *Facilitated Communication* has recently had a considerable impact on teaching children with autism in North America. In this technique, the child's hand is held over a computer keyboard by the adult (the 'facilitator'), and under such physical guidance it is reported that the children communicate more easily. In the *Option Process*, developed by Barry and Suzi Kauffman, volunteers make a 24-hour commitment to intensive work on developing a relationship with the child, while parents are encouraged to join a family programme. Finally, in the *Camphill Communities*, and their schools and villages, some children and adults with autism are given places alongside others with a mental handicap. These schools, colleges, and villages run along principles developed by Rudolph Steiner, encourage communal values and working in nature, and provide individual attention. These schools are less structured than those run by the National Autistic Society.

These psychological therapies are exciting in that they represent the continuing inspiration with which clinicians are trying to overcome key symptoms in autism; but they are also somewhat difficult to assess, as they have often had no independent evaluation of the sometimes considerable claims their proponents make. As with all claims for cures, parents should be cautious. Cures will hopefully come one day, and the way we will recognize a cure will be after 'blind' assessors (i.e. assessors who do not know which kind of treatment a child has received) compare children who have been treated with similarly diagnosed children of the same mental age who have not received that treatment.

10.

Medical treatments

I have the dream that one day they will develop a wonder-drug that will allow his brain to work properly again. But could it really be that simple?

Drug treatments for autism

With the realization that biological factors are of fundamental importance in causing autism, the search for drug treatments has gained ground. As yet, there is no drug which clearly leads to improvements in the basic symptoms of autism. As with psychological treatments, it is important, therefore, to be cautious in accepting claims to the contrary. This does not mean, however, that drugs are of no use in treating certain aspects of autism. A number of drugs have been tried as treatments, and the evidence for their effectiveness is briefly outlined below.

● *Fenfluramine*
Fenfluramine is a drug that reduces the blood level of *serotonin*. Serotonin is a natural chemical that has been found to be high in about a third of children with autism. When fenfluramine was first used in the United States there was great excitement, with claims that it was a 'wonder drug' for autism. Since then, it has been recognized that these early claims were wildly optimistic. It now seems more likely that fenfluramine has few if any clearly beneficial effects. The change in opinion occurred following 'blind' trials (in which doctors evaluate the child's behaviour *without knowing* which medication the child is on). Although fenfluramine has not been found to produce unwanted side-effects in people, there is evidence to suggest that it can damage the nervous system in animals. At present, therefore, this must be considered an experimental treatment that should only be embarked upon under specialist medical supervision in recognized centres.

● *Megavitamins*
Exceptionally high doses of vitamin B_6 in conjunction with magnesium have been advocated as a treatment for autism. This treatment has been

advocated on the basis of reports of improvements and on the basis that large doses of vitamin B_6 are not associated with known side-effects. However, when vitamin B_6 treatment is stopped there can be increased disturbance, and this *withdrawal effect* may be mistakenly taken as evidence for the effectiveness of the medication. In addition, while unwanted side-effects from vitamin B_6 are rare, there is evidence for unwanted side-effects from other medicines that the person may be taking in conjunction with vitamin B_6 (such as magnesium, or large doses of other vitamins, or anti-epileptic medication). For these reasons we recommend that megavitamin treatment should also only be used under specialist medical supervision, and currently only as an experimental treatment.

● *Major tranquillizers*
The term 'major tranquillizer' refers to a number of different but related drugs (such as haloperidol, chlorpromazine, and thioridazine) that are frequently used in the treatment of adults with psychiatric disorders. They are sometimes used for children with autism, not because they improve the autism itself, but because they can provide temporary relief from agitation, aggression, insomnia, stereotypies (repetitive behaviours), or other behaviour problems. They are very powerful drugs, and can produce unwanted side-effects, especially if used over a long period. Fortunately, many of these side-effects reverse on stopping the treatment; but occasionally neurological problems may develop as a result of the medication, and these can be irreversible. For these reasons these drugs are mainly used to help break a maladaptive style of behaviour, or as a temporary adjunct to other forms of treatment.

● *Naltrexone*
This drug acts by blocking the effects of naturally occurring substances called *opioids* that are found in the brain. At present the drug is being evaluated for its effectiveness in the treatment of autism, and until these studies are completed it should be regarded as an experimental form of treatment that is not appropriate for routine use.

Drug treatments for epilepsy

Epilepsy occurs in up to 30 per cent of children with autism. It may take many forms, ranging from full blown seizures to 'absence attacks', in which the person seems to 'blank out' for a few seconds or minutes. Epilepsy in autism sometimes does not begin until adolescence. In some instances, individuals may develop more than one type of seizure. The standard procedures for assessing and treating anyone with epilepsy are equally applicable to a person with autism who develops seizures. Thus, a detailed evaluation (including an EEG and sometimes a brain scan) and anti-convulsant medication, with regular monitoring of blood levels, may be required. But, as a rule, if the child (or adult) has just one or two fits, treatment may not be needed, unless the fits recur. If they do recur, the usual cautions apply to prevent the person from injuring him or herself during an attack. (For more information on this, the reader can consult a companion volume in this series, *Epilepsy: the facts*.) If medical treatment controls the seizures, and if there is no recurrence of a fit for several years, a trial period of withdrawing the medication may be attempted. Such a period is helpful in identifying those people in whom epilepsy spontaneously disappears. Psychological treatments for epilepsy may also be needed, if for example assessment reveals that stress or other factors increase the risk of attacks.

Other issues in the treatment of autism

Health promotion

Medical knowledge about healthy living is as relevant to people with autism as to anyone else. Thus, a balanced diet and regular exercise should be one goal. In addition, regular health and dental check-ups should take place. This is particularly important for people with autism, because their ability to identify medical and dental problems and communicate that they are experiencing them may be severely limited. For example, if they lack speech, problems such as severe toothache, headache, ear infections, etc., may only become apparent because they begin to injure themselves, or develop increasingly disturbed behaviour.

It is also important to ensure that the people who are responsible for the care of people with autism remain healthy. This is particularly important in view of the stresses associated with the care of any disabled person. Parents and siblings need to be careful to ensure that their needs do not get relegated or minimized, and professionals should arrange additional support in the form of respite care, holiday breaks, and home-helps.

Alternative treatments

Drugs for the treatment of *Candida* infections, and various alternative therapies (for example homoeopathy and cranial osteopathy) have been advocated for the treatment of autism. None of these treatments have been shown to be effective, although mainstream medical practitioners have often not formally evaluated these therapies. Many of them are not in themselves harmful, and in some instances beneficial effects may result from changes in the parents' sense of involvement in the therapy. However, whatever changes these therapies do produce, there is no evidence that they amount to a cure. Systematic and independent evaluation of treatment has been emphasized in this chapter because of the dangers of unsystematic appraisal of therapies. Unsystematic appraisal may lead to parents' hopes being raised unrealistically. Hope must be based on reasonable evidence.

11.

Adolescence and adulthood

In many ways it was easier when he was younger. Of course he was just as odd then as he is now, but it was somehow easier to accept in a child—lots of children do odd things. Now he is older he seems to stand out more as different, and that is still difficult for me to cope with. But I have become that much better at explaining to people what is wrong with him; I am stronger than in those early days, better at finding solutions, and more realistic.

In this chapter we consider the range of outcomes that usually occur in people with autism, to give a sense of what can be expected. This by no means defines the limits, but nevertheless summarizes the kinds of outcomes we have seen in our clinic. Following this we look at specific issues relating to adjustment in adolescence and early adulthood.

Typical outcomes in autism

Currently, our knowledge is limited by the fact that very few studies have followed people with autism into their later adult life, and by the fact that elderly people known to have autism are rare, since the disorder itself was only identified in the middle of this century. We do know, however, that the range of outcomes is very wide. Thus, for people with autism who also have severe mental handicap, some sort of life-long support and supervision will be essential. For more able individuals, outcome really depends on how much useful language the person has acquired. As a common-sense rule, the less language a person has, the more support he or she will need. It is however important to note that language can develop even as late as adolescence, although the rate of development by this age may be slow and limited.

For the most able people with autism, a life of independence and employment in the open market-place is not unknown; but this is unusual. Sheltered accommodation and employment is more usual. Other options include day centres, in which the individual is given interesting activities and some training, but may not be employed. Some issues surrounding employment and placement are discussed later. It is worth noting that currently almost three-quarters of people with autism require a residential sheltered placement.

Problems in adolescence

Adolescence is a time when all children change, both physically and emotionally. Naturally, the changes one sees in people with autism are different to those in other people. Normal adolescents, for example, often rebel in different ways against their parents, and spend increasingly more time away from them. In autism, these changes do not occur to the same degree, and may not occur at all. In some adolescents with autism, improvement in their social understanding is seen, and this can make life much easier, because more can be communicated. Occasionally, the other side of this coin is that some adolescents with autism begin to get a dawning realization that they are different from other people, that unlike others of their age they are not finding girl- or boyfriends, going out independently, or able to think of having an independent future. This can lead to occasional depression, for which help may need to be sought.

The physical changes of puberty are no different in adolescents with autism from other adolescents, but their understanding of their sexuality is often rather more limited. Sex education may be needed in order to reduce the risk of exploitation either of others or by others, and in order to explain to a person with autism when and where activities such as kissing or masturbation are acceptable, and when and where they are not. Some adolescents and adults with autism do desire sexual relationships, but frequently do not understand how to develop such a relationship. This problem can be approached as part of a broader social skills training programme to help the person learn about different kinds of friendship. There are a range of educational materials available to aid sex education, and such materials, though designed for care-staff, may also be valuable for parents to use, in that it is often parents who 'discover' their child's sexuality at home, and worry about how to react.

Deterioration in puberty

There are some worrying reports of an *overall decline* or deterioration in a small minority of people with autism that occurs during puberty and after. While the majority of people with autism fortunately continue to learn and develop both intellectually and in other ways, well into adulthood, some do sadly get worse. This can be seen in a slowing down in learning, and in the fact that IQ test scores become slightly lower; and in a proportion of people, in the onset of epilepsy, which occurs for the first time in their lives at this stage. These changes, it should be stressed, only occur in a minority of people; but if it is your child, it is naturally a massive disappointment. After all the years of hoping for improvement, and indeed after seeing real gains, a decline in skills is a blow. For these few people, renewed consultation with specialists may be needed, especially if convulsions are repeating, in which case medication is needed. Thankfully, most cases of epilepsy in autism are treatable with such medication. Most adolescents, however, do not show deterioration, and the worry instead becomes: how can the intensive support and educational benefit that was coming from the school continue when he or she leaves school?

Issues in residential placement and employment

At present, provision of services for adults with autism is still wholly insufficient. This is true both in the areas of sheltered residences and sheltered employment, as well as in occupational training. The worst effect of the lack of opportunities is that all the years of high-quality education can be undone by the relative lack of stimulation in adulthood. Despite this clear lack of sufficient resources, it is important to summarize what sorts of provision are currently considered worth aiming for.

In the area of residential care, models include small group homes, designed to be as much like any other person's home as possible, to avoid the problems of institutionalization and stigmatization; these might be for four or six people, with one or two care staff living in the same home. Such homes are ideally indistinguishable from and as much a part of the local community as possible. Other models include larger sheltered communities, which may be in towns or in rural areas, but in which work and leisure opportunities are located on the same site as the residences. Such larger sheltered communities often work extremely well, but risk leaving the residents somewhat isolated from the wider community. There is no doubt that these settings have overcome the worst aspects of earlier forms of institutionalization (such as poor décor, lack of privacy, and degrading practices), but they nevertheless suffer one drawback over the smaller model of housing mentioned earlier, in that they make autism conspicuous to other people. Such a drawback needs to be considered alongside the obvious advantages of the often beautiful farm or market-garden settings of such places, and the fact that residents are less exposed to the hazards of life in the open community.

In the area of employment up to now relatively little has been achieved, and similar issues arise. Work currently tends to be either rather limited in scope (some employers taking on people with autism to do rather repetitive jobs, often below the person's full potential), or is only found in the larger sheltered communities mentioned above, where activities such as crafts, farming, and gardening are encouraged, often to quite a high level. An exciting philosophy being put into practice in a few centres now (such as those in New Haven, USA) is the idea that in principle there is no limit to the sorts of industries or professional workplaces a person with autism could work in, given adequate support from a key worker. This approach is exciting because it shatters the myth that the only jobs people with autism can do are low-level and repetitive ones, such as stacking shelves in supermarkets.

Is this a pipe-dream? Such optimism is already producing results in some places. For example, people with autism are finding work in lawyers' offices, doing highly valued clerical duties, or are working in bicycle-repair shops, demonstrating technical expertise, or are working in children's crèches, in a gentle and responsible way, or are playing jazz in cafés, bringing pleasure to many others. Such successful integration into the open job-market is usually the result of painstaking efforts behind the scenes by key workers, reassuring employers that autism is not a threatening or dangerous condition, and that odd tantrums or strange behaviour do not represent real obstacles to doing the job, and explaining that strange behaviour often only occurs as a reaction to unexpected changes in work routines.

If employers can be persuaded to accept the person's autism, and to support the principle of equal opportunities for people with disabilities, then we will hopefully see an expansion of such jobs. In the USA, tax incentives to employers are encouraging this trend. Ultimately, social attitudes will determine how successful such employment is. The goal of widening occupational opportunities naturally has more chance of success for more able people with autism. However, in principle, opportunities at the right level should be available for less able people with autism too. Just because a person lacks language, this need not prevent them from being able to hold down a job, given the right training. This is a challenge for the future.

Appendix 1:

International societies and associations for children and adults with autism

We are very grateful to Tessa Hall, Information Officer of the National Autistic Society (UK) who compiled the information below. Further details can be obtained from her directly.

AUTISM EUROPE
The International Association Autism Europe
rue Emile Leger 4
B-1495 Villers-la-Ville
Belgium
(Tel: 32 (0) 71 87 95 94)

ARGENTINA
Centro de Atención Integral Para Niños Autista y Psicoticos
Santiago Del Estero 239
4400 Salta Argentina
(Tel.: 211326)

AUSTRALIA
National Association for Autism (Australia)
PO Box 339
Eastwood
South Australia 5063

The Autistic Children's Association of Queensland (Inc.)
437, Hellawell Road
PO Box 363
Sunnybank
Queensland 4109
Australia

Association for Autistic Children in Western Australia
Suite 114
396, Scarborough Beach Road
Osborne Park
Western Australia 6017

Society for Autistic Children in Tasmania
17 Sunshine Road
Austins Ferry
T 7011
Australia

The Autistic Children's Association of South Australia (Inc.)
3 Fisher Street
Myrtle Bank
South Australia 5064
(Tel.: 79 6976)

Autistic Association of NSW
41 Cook Street
Forestville
NSW 2087, Australia
(Tel.: (02) 452 4041)

Victorian Autistic Children's and Adults' Association
P.O. Box 235
Ashburton 3147
Victoria
Australia
(Tel.: (03) 885 0533)

AUSTRIA
Osterreichischer Verein Zur Hilfe fur Autisten
A-1010 Wien
Esslinggasse 13/3/11
Austria
(Tel: 53 39 666)

BELGIUM
Association De Parents Pour Epanouissement Des Personnes Autistes *
Rue J. Stallaert, 1 bte 4
B-1060 Bruxelles
Belgique
(Tel.: +32 2 344 56 87)

Opleidingscentrum Autisme *
Laar 61
B-2140 Antwerpen-Borgerhout
Belgique
(Tel.: +32 3 235 37 55)

Vlaamse Vereniging Autisme *
Groot Begijnhof, 14
B-9040 Gent
Belgique
(Tel.: +32 (91) 28 98 79)

BRAZIL
Associacão de Protecão Aos Autistas
Av. Robert Kennedy
3345 - Interlagos, CEP 04772
São Paulo, Brasil
(Tel.: 246.4718)

Associacão Brasileira de Autismo
Sector de Divulgacão e Publicãoes
Estrada Da Canoa 401
S. Conrado (22610)
Rio de Janeiro
Brasil

Associacão de Amigos do Autista
Av. Ipiransa 919
16. andar cj. 1606
01039 São Paulo, Brasil

BULGARIA
Parent's Association Autistic Child, Sofia *
c/o President: Mrs Anny Baltova
1000 Sofia
Oboriste 21
Bulgaria
(Tel.: 44 47 16)

CANADA
Autism Society Canada
129 Yorkville Avenue
Suite 202
Toronto, Ontario
Canada M5R 1C4
(Tel.: 416 922 0302)

CHILE
Asociación de Padres y Amigos de los Autistas
(Quinta Región)
Vina del Mar
7 Norte 544
Casilla 844, Chile

CROATIA
Croatian Society for Helping Autistic Persons *
Dvorniciceva 6
41000 Zagreb
Croatia
(Tel.: 38.41.33.4)

DENMARK
*Psykotiske Borns vel Landsforeningen for Autister**
48, Skovvejen
8740 Braedstrup
Denmark
(Tel.: 45.75.28.18)

FINLAND
*Finnish Association for Autism** *(Interessforeningen for Bar Barndomspsykoser**)*
Stenbackinkatu 7A
SF-00250 Helsinki, Finland
(Tel.: (358) 0414 373)

FRANCE *(See also* Reunion Islands)
*Association de Parents et Professionnels Pour L'education, le Developpement,
L'integration Des Personnes Atteintes D'autisme**
2, rue Albert de Mun, bat.3
F-92190 Meudon
France

*Autisme—Ile de France**
52, rue du Docteur Blanche
F-75016 Paris
France
(Tel.: + 33 1 45 25 82 52)

*Pro Aid Autism**
84, rue Didot
F-75014 Paris
France
(Tel.: +33 1 45 45 72 59)

*Sesame Autisme**
18, rue Etex
F-75018 Paris
France
(Tel.: +33 1 42 28 57 09)

*Union Nationale des Associations de Parents et Amis de Personnes Handicapees
Mentales**
Rue Coysevox, 15
F-75018 Paris
France
(Tel.: +33 1 42 63 84 33)

GERMANY
*Bundesverband Hilfe für das Autistische Kind**
Bebelallee 141
D-2000 Hamburg 60
Germany
(Tel.: 49 (0) 40 5 11 56 04)

GREAT BRITAIN
*National Autistic Society**
276, Willesden Lane
London NW2 5RB
(Tel.: 081-451-1114)

The Scottish Society for Autistic Children
24d Barony Street
Edinburgh
Lothian EH3 6NY
(Tel.: 031-557-0474)

GREECE
Society of Parents and Friends of Autistic Children
14 Kanari Street
Alimos 174 55
Greece
(Tel.: 98.37.090)

HONG KONG
Society for the Welfare of the Autistic Persons
Room 210-14
Block 19
Shek Kip Mei Estate
Kowloon, Hong Kong
(Tel.: 7883326)

HUNGARY
*Autism Foundation Hungary**
Dr. Anna Balazz
Budapest 1X, Taviro U.21
1098 Hungary
(Tel.: +36 17 1213 526 Ex.55)

ICELAND
*Umsjonarfelag Einhverfra**
Postholf 4148
Posthof
IS - 104 Reykjavik
Iceland

INDIA
Autistic Society of India
c/o *TAMANA*
183, Munirka Enclave
New Delhi - 110067
India

IRELAND
Irish Society for Autism *
Unity Building
16/17 Lower O'Connell Street
Dublin 1
Eire
(Tel.: 353 1 744684)

ISRAEL
Israeli Society for Autistic Children
PO Box 32097
Tel Aviv 61320
Israel
(Tel.: 03-234965)

ITALY
ANFFAS Gruppo Autismo e Psicosi *
Via C. Bazzi, 68
I-20142 Milano
Italie
(Tel.: +39.2.84.63.406 - 84.33.773)

Associazione Nazionale Genitori Soggeti Autistici *
Casella Postale no. 3102
I-40131 Bologna
Italie
(Tel.: +39.51 63.43.367)

Associazione Parenti e Amici Psicottici e Autistici *
c/o Scuola Amerigo Vespucci
Via Bolognese 238
I-50139 Firenze
Italie
(Tel.: +39.56.40.05.94)

*Associazione Per La Ricerca Italiana Sulla Sindrome Di Down, L'autismo e
il Danno Cerebrale* *
c/o ANFFAS
Via Rasi, 14
I-Bologna
Italie
(Tel.: +39.51.24.95.72)

JAPAN
The Autism Society Japan
c/o Zenkoku Fukushi Zaidan Centre
2-2-8 Nishi-Waseda
Shinjuku-ku
Tokyo, 162
Japan

LUXEMBOURG
Association Luxembourgeoise d'Aide aux personnes autistiques *
33 rue Antoine Meyer
L-2153 Luxembourg
(Tel.: (00352) 458009)

MALAYSIA
National Autistic Society of Malaysia
Fakulti Psikiatri
Universiti Kebangsaan Malaysia
Jalan Raja Muda
Kuala Lumpur
Malaysia

MEXICO
Centro Educativo Domas, AC
Calzada de la Viga 1225
Colonia Marte
Mexico, D.F.
08830

Centro de Rehabilitación y Educación Especial
(CREE) Mérida, Yuc
Col. Francisco I. Madero
Mérida, Yucatan
Mexico

NETHERLANDS
Nederlandse Vereniging voor autisme en verwante contactstoornissen *
Postbus 1367
1400 BJ Bussum
Netherlands
(Tel.: (02159) 31557)

NEW ZEALAND
Autistic Association of NZ
c/o Mr. R. Belton (President)
52 Leinster Avenue
Raumati South
New Zealand

Autistic Children's Sub-committee, NZ Society for the Intellectually Handicapped
5 Buchanan Street
Wellington 1
New Zealand

NORWAY
*Landsforeningen for autister**
PB 118, Ksjelsaas
n-04 11 Oslo
Norway
(Tel.: 47.2.180 923)

PANAMA
Panamanian Society for the Parents of Autistic Children
Apartado 6
141 - Zona 6
El Dorado
Panama

POLAND
Krajowe Towarzystwo Autyzmu
Stawki 5/7
00-183 Warsaw
Poland

Stowarzyszenie Pomocy Osobom Autystycznym w Gdansku
ulica Kosciuszki 91. 4
80-421 Gdansk
Poland

Autistic Society of Lower Silesia
53-621 Wroclaw
Glogowska St.
30
Poland

PORTUGAL
*Associacāo Portuguesa para Proteccāo aos Deficientes Autistas**
218, r/c Rua de Junqueira
1300 Lisboa, Portugal
(Tel.: 351.1.63.85.67)

REUNION ISLANDS (*See also* France)
Autisme Reunion
Nathalie Faucher
42 Route Des Palmiers
97417 La Montagne
Reunion Islands

RUSSIA
*Dobro Association for Autistic Children Care**
Kazarmenny per., 4 str.apart. 1-2
109028 Moscow
Russia
(Tel.: +7.095.238.97.37)

SINGAPORE
The Autistic Association (Singapore)
Eddie Koh Swee Hua (Chairman)
c/o Block 97C Upper
Thomson Road #05-10
Lakeview Estate
Singapore 2057

SOUTH AFRICA
Association for Autism (SAASSPER)
PO Box 35833
Menlopark
Pretoria, 0102
South Africa
(Tel.: 012-47-27820)

South African Society for Autistic Children
Private Bag X4
Clareinch 7740
Cape Town 8001
South Africa

Society for Children & Adults with Autism
PO Box 87190
Houghton
Johannesburg
2041 South Africa

SPAIN
Associacio de Pares amb Fills autistes *
3 Carrer Puigblanc
Mataro (Catalunya), Espagna
(Tel.: 34.3.790.31.55)

Associacio de Pares amb Fills autistes i caracterials de Catalunya (APAFACC) *
Ave. san Antonio-Maria Claret,
282 A 2n2a,
Barcelona 08026, Espagna
(Tel.: 34.3.235.16.79)

Associacion Guipuzoana de Autismo y Psichosis infantiles (GAUTENA) *
Avenida de Francia 5
Apartado 1000
20080 San Sebastián, Espagna
(Tel.: 34.4.321.53.44)

Associacio del Centre Especialitza de reducicio d'autistes i caracterials *
Ave. San Antonio-Maria Claret
282 A 2n2a
Barcelona 08026, Espagna
(Tel.: 34.3.23.51.679)

Associacion espanola de padres de ninos autistos (APNA) *
9 Navaleno
28033
Madrid, Espagna
(Tel.: 34.1.76.62.222)

Associacion Espanola de Padres de ninos Autistos de Burgos *
Calle Les Torres, s/n
SP 09007, Burgos
Espagna
(Tel.: 34.2.39.142)

SWEDEN
Riksforeningen Autism *
Bondegatan 1D
116 23 Stockholm, Sweden
(Tel.: 46.8.702.0580)

SWITZERLAND
*L'Association Suisse de Parents d'Enfants Autistes et de Personnes Intéressées
par l'Autisme* *
'Secretariat d'information et de documentation sur les problèmes de l'autisme'
21 rue St Pierre Canisius
1700 Fribourg, Switzerland
(Tel.: 037 21 97 88)

TRINIDAD and TOBAGO
Autistic Society of Trinidad & Tobago
c/o Mr. M. Copeland (Vice-President)
25 Altyre Drive, Cocoyea
San Fernando
Trinidad
West Indies
(Tel.: 653-3708)

TURKEY
Ilgi Society to Protect Autistic Children
17.Sok.47/2
Bahcelievler
Ankara
Turkey

UNITED STATES OF AMERICA
Autism Society of America Inc.
8601 Georgia Avenue
Suite 503
Silver Spring
MD 20910
USA
(Tel.: (301) 565-0433)

URUGUAY
The Uruguayan Autistic Children Parents' Association
Enrique Martínez 1195
Montevideo
Uruguay

VENEZUELA
Parents Association for Autistic Children
Apartado 3455
Caracas
Venezuela

(* Member associations: Autisme Europe = 34)

(September 1993).

Appendix 2:

Two systems used by psychiatrists for diagnosing autism

1. The DSM-III-R criteria for autism (the American Diagnostic Scheme)

At least eight of the following sixteen items are present, these to include at least two items from A, one from B, and one from C.

A. Qualitative impairment in reciprocal social interaction. As shown by:

- Marked lack of awareness of the existence or feelings of others (e.g., treats a person as if he/she were a piece of the furniture; does not notice the distress of another person; apparently has no concept of the need of others for privacy).

- No or abnormal seeking of comfort at times of distress (e.g., does not come for comfort even when ill, hurt or tired; seeks comfort in a stereo-typed way, e.g., says 'cheese' when hurt).

- No or impaired imitation (e.g., does not wave bye-bye; does not copy mother's domestic activities; mechanical imitation of others' actions out of context).

- No or abnormal social play (e.g., does not actively participate in simple games; prefers solitary play activities; involves other children in play only as 'mechanical aids').

- Gross impairment in ability to make peer friendships (e.g., no interest in making peer friendships; despite interest in making friends, demonstrates lack of understanding of conventions of social interaction, for example reads phone book to uninterested peer).

B. Qualitative impairment in verbal and non-verbal communication, and in imaginative activity. As shown by:

- No mode of communication, such as communicative babbling, facial expression, gesture, mime, or spoken language.

- Markedly abnormal non-verbal communication, as in the use of eye gaze, facial expression, body posture or gesture to initiate or modulate social interaction (e.g., does not anticipate being held, stiffens when held, does not look at the person or smile when making a social approach, does not greet parents or visitors, has a fixed stare in social situations).

- Absence of imaginative activity, such as play-acting of adult roles, fantasy characters, or animals; lack of interest in stories about imaginary events.

- Marked abnormalities in the production of speech, including volume, pitch, stress, rate, rhythm, and intonation (e.g., monotonous tone, question-like melody, or high pitch).

- Marked abnormalities in the form or content of speech, including stereotyped and repetitive use of speech (e.g., immediate echolalia or mechanical repetition of television commercial); use of 'you' when 'I' is meant (e.g., using 'you want a cookie?' to mean 'I want a cookie'); idiosyncratic use of words or phrases (e.g., 'Go on green riding' to mean 'I want to go on the swing'); or frequent irrelevant remarks (e.g., starts talking about train schedules during a conversation about sports).

- Marked impairment in the ability to initiate or sustain conversation with others, despite adequate speech (e.g., indulging in lengthy monologues on one subject regardless of interjections from others).

C. Markedly restricted repertoire of activities and interests, as shown by:

- Stereotyped bodily movements, e.g., hand flicking or twisting, spinning, head-banging, complex whole body movements.

- Persistent preoccupation with parts of objects (e.g., sniffing or smelling objects, repetitive feeling of textures of materials, spinning wheels of toy cars) or attachment to unusual objects (e.g., insists on carrying around a piece of string).

- Marked distress over changes in trivial aspects of environment, (e.g., when a vase is moved from its usual position).

- Unreasonable insistence on following routines in precise detail, (e.g., insisting that exactly the same route always be followed when shopping).

- Markedly restricted range of interests and a preoccupation with one narrow interest, (e.g., interested only in lining objects, in amassing facts about meteorology, or in pretending to be a fantasy character).

D. Specify if onset during infancy or childhood (after 36 months).

2. The ICD-10 system *

- Presence of abnormal/impaired development before 3 years of age.

- Qualitative impairments in reciprocal social interaction (3 from the following 5 areas):
  - Failure to use eye gaze, body posture, facial expression, and gesture to regulate interaction adequately.
  - A failure to develop (in a manner appropriate to mental age, and despite ample opportunity) peer relationships that involve a mutual sharing of interests, activities, and emotions.
  - Rarely seeking and using other people for comfort and affection at times of stress or distress and/or offering comfort and affection to others when they are showing distress or unhappiness.
  - A lack of shared enjoyment in terms of vicarious pleasures in other people's happiness and/or a spontaneous seeking to share their own enjoyment through joint involvement with others.
  - A lack of socioemotional reciprocity, as shown by an impaired or deviant response to other people's emotions; and/or lack of modulation of behaviour according to the social context; and/or a weak integration of socioemotional and communicative behaviours.

- Qualitative impairments in communication (2 from the following 5 areas):
  - A delay in, or total lack of, spoken language that is not accompanied by an attempt to compensate through the use of gesture or mime as alternative modes of communication.
  - A relative failure to initiate or sustain conversational interchange (at whatever level of language skills is present) in which there is reciprocal to-and-fro responsiveness to the communication of the other person.
  - Stereotyped and repetitive use of language and/or idiosyncratic use of words or phrases.
  - Abnormalities in pitch, stress, rate, rhythm, and intonation of speech.
  - A lack of varied spontaneous make-believe play, or, when young, social imitative play.

---

* Adapted from an early draft of the ICD-10 classification of mental and behavioural disorders: draft criteria for research. WHO, Geneva. (In press.)

- Restricted, repetitive, and stereotyped patterns of behaviour, interests, and activities (2 from the following 6 areas):

  - An encompassing preoccupation with stereotyped and restricted patterns of interest.
  - Specific attachments to unusual objects.
  - Apparently compulsive adherence to specific, non-functional routines or rituals.
  - Stereotyped and repetitive motor mannerisms that involve either hand/finger flapping or twisting or complex whole-body movements.
  - Preoccupation with part-objects or non-functional elements of play materials (such as odour, the feel of their surface, or the noise/vibration that they generate).
  - Distress over changes in small, non-functional details of the environment.

- Clinical picture is not attributable to other varieties of pervasive developmental disorder; specific developmental disorder of receptive language with secondary socioemotional problems; reactive attachment disorder or disinhibited attachment disorder; mental retardation with some associated emotional/behavioural disorder; schizophrenia of unusually early onset; and Rett's syndrome.

Appendix 3:

Some examples of behaviour therapy for specific problems

Parents often hope there will be a quick recipe for solving a behaviour problem, and while this is sometimes the case, treatments for specific problems in autism usually need careful and individual consideration. As a first port of call, parents in the UK can always telephone the National Autistic Society Helpline (or its equivalent in other countries), in case one of their 'handy tips' is useful. Otherwise, the National Autistic Society can send a relevant booklet which deals with the particular category of behaviour difficulty, if this is available. In Britain, these booklets include those compiled by the Association of Principals of National Autistic Society and Local Autistic Society Schools and Units. For example, one recently completed booklet (1991) of theirs on *Managing feeding difficulties in children with autism* describes a wide range of different eating problems and how to approach their management. A comprehensive review of these methods is beyond the scope of the present book. Instead, we describe a few of the techniques used for some selected and common behaviour problems; but these should be thought of only as a starting-point towards more detailed advice and help.

Toileting difficulties

Incontinence can represent a major problem in some children with autism. Careful assessment of the causes of the wetting or soiling is important. For example, it may result from a delay in the acquisition of bladder and bowel control, in which case toilet-training may be helpful. For night-wetting, a method such as the 'bell and pad' may be appropriate. The bell and pad can be obtained from a child psychologist or psychiatrist, and literally involves a bell which rings automatically whenever the child begins to become incontinent. This simple device helps the child to learn to anticipate when to ask for or go to the toilet. Behavioural programmes such as 'star charts', in which stars (or other rewarding items) are used to reward dry periods of the day or night, may be implemented by a psychologist in conjunction with those caring for the person with autism. Such programmes need to be carefully tailored to the individual, and parents should ask to be referred to a specialist clinic.

A few children with autism develop the habit of smearing faeces, and this needs a clear and consistent behaviour programme (rewarding him or her for not doing it) if the child fails to learn its unacceptability. Advice from a psychologist should be sought at the earliest stage, as the lack of hygiene associated with this behaviour naturally carries health risks, both for the child with autism and for others living in the same home.

Aggression

Fortunately most people with autism do not show excessive aggression, although they naturally show anger, just as other people do, at times of frustration. Nevertheless, certain kinds of aggression are sometimes seen in children with autism. Often these take the form of the person hitting or in some other way hurting another person; but questioning often reveals that the person often was unaware of the emotional impact this might have on the 'victim', even though they may have been very aware of the physical effects on them (such as making them cry). Teaching them about the other person's feelings may be worth trying; but usually a more direct and simple method will involve rewarding alternative, non-aggressive behaviour. Again, a psychologist should be consulted to help to achieve this.

Preoccupations and repetitive behaviours

Obsessive behaviour is one of the key characteristics of autism. Should it be 'removed', simply because it is unusual? By itself, its unusual quality is an insufficient reason to warrant treatment. After all, we all have unusual aspects to our personality, and we have the right to be ourselves, complete with our eccentricities. However, if the obsession is in some way impeding the person's development, then treatment might be considered.

For example, John (in Chapter 1), when he was ten years old, would only read alphabet books, and no other ones. In a real sense, this was limiting his educational development. In circumstances such as these, the particular preoccupations can be broadened or even overcome completely, by focusing on other behaviours (for example, reading other books) and rewarding these each time, whilst gradually reducing the amount of time the person is allowed to engage in his or her obsession. Notice, however, that what is changed is not the obsessionality itself, but merely the behaviour. Evidence that this is the case is seen in the fact that children with autism often develop new preoccupations when earlier ones are overcome, and sometimes they 'revert' to old routines at particular times.

Embarrassing behaviour

Doing embarrassing things is another sign of the social naïveté of many children with autism. When it occurs, it is not 'wilful' or 'deliberate', as some people might at first think, nor is it 'designed to annoy me', as many parents might imagine. It is simply a reflection of the severe inability most people with autism have in appreciating other people's thoughts and feelings. Examples of embarrassing behaviour that are commonly reported to occur in autism are of the person saying the 'wrong' thing at the wrong time (for instance, truthfully commenting that the head-teacher's grey hair now looks blacker); or doing the 'wrong' thing at the wrong time (such as rubbing their genitals conspicuously during the school Christmas party); or simply being oblivious of the social norms which implicitly govern particular situations (for example, staring at people on the train). Teaching the 'right' way of behaving can only be done at the time the embarrassing behaviour occurs, and usually needs to be done with each example of such behaviours. It is an example of how social skills training needs intensive individual work, simply because for people with autism such sensitivity to social cues does not come naturally.

Self-injury

The most effective treatment for self-injury, such as head-banging, biting, and hitting oneself, is based on a careful evaluation of the factors triggering the self-injury, and the factors maintaining it. Behaviour therapy is the most useful form of intervention. Protective devices, such as helmets, arm-splints, and gloves are also sometimes used temporarily to prevent severe damage to the head or body, and until the self-injury has been controlled by psychological intervention. Self-injury is distressing for others to witness, as well as for the person engaged in it. It is important, though not easy, for both care staff and family members to all respond consistently in implementing the behaviour programme to treat the self-injury, if it is to succeed. So, for example, if assessment of the self-injury reveals that it is maintained by, among other things, the attention the person receives through doing it, the behaviour programme may require other family members and care staff to literally turn away from the person when the self-injury begins, and only provide attention during periods of non-injury.

Such a response runs counter to our natural reaction of wanting to help and reassure the person during self-injury, and may therefore be very difficult to carry out. However, a consistent behaviour programme is the only way to establish if that factor, such as attention, is indeed the cause. Once the cause has been identified, teaching the person alternative strategies other than self-injury can begin. Thus, to take another common cause of self-injury, if a person without speech is head-banging in order to 'escape' from a difficult task, they can be taught to signal in some other way that they wish to have a rest from the task. Self-injury in most cases is treatable through such techniques, but rare cases do exist in which the behaviours do not diminish even though the programmes have been strictly followed. In all cases of self-injury, behaviour programmes need to be followed under the direction of an experienced clinician.

Eating difficulties
Pica, or eating and swallowing inedible substances such as earth, stones, glass, and paint, can be problematic. A physical examination should be carried out in order to check if medical conditions (such as iron deficiency, lead poisoning, or zinc deficiency) are causing it, and in order to check if complications (such as intestinal damage, obstruction, or infestation) have developed. Treatment of such associated medical conditions, including iron supplements, can then be implemented, and may lead to a reduction in the behaviour. Otherwise, behavioural treatments, based on rewarding the eating of edible substances, are most appropriate.

Aside from pica, another common type of eating difficulty is excessive, fussy eating. For example, some children with autism will only eat certain foods, and others will only eat food if it is always arranged in exactly the same way on the plate. This may represent one instance of a person's obsessive, ritualistic behaviour. Such obsessive styles of eating are often maintained simply because parents and others want to avoid the tantrum they know will follow if the food is not prepared according to their child's wishes. Such a response by parents is entirely understandable. However, at times such inflexible eating habits are impossible to satisfy, and so it is worth attempting to change the child's eating behaviour towards greater flexibility at the earliest opportunity.

Some ways of achieving this include general introduction of minute quantities of foods that the child is refusing to eat, or gradual and minute changes in the arrangement of the food, until a range of foods or arrangements are tolerated. The alternative approach is to implement a big change quickly, and then weather the tantrum this may provoke. Once the child discovers that his or her tantrums do not bring a return of the favourite food or plate, the tantrums may eventually subside. This is especially likely if the child is hungry! But caution is required, as occasional attempts at 'self-starvation' have been seen.

Tantrums

Tantrums, whether they are caused by disturbing rigid eating patterns or other preoccupations, do eventually diminish as a result of literally leaving the person to learn that nothing is being gained by the tantrum. Parents and others often worry that the tantrum will get out of control and that the person may suffer some self-inflicted injury. In this situation parents and other carers should ensure that the person has a safe place to have his or her tantrum: moving chairs and other furniture with sharp corners to the edge of the room, or moving the person into an emptier space such as a hallway or spare room, can remove the anxiety of risk of injury, while not 'giving in' to the tantrum. In this way, tantrums should eventually subside. It is important that someone should be present during a tantrum to ensure that no injury or damage is done. A useful and effective additional technique is so-called 'passive restraint', where carers are taught to hold the person in such a way that no one is physically injured.

For further advice on behaviour therapy, parents should ask their GP to refer them to their local health visitor or clinical psychologist.

Recommended further reading

For an excellent account of current psychological research in autism, see *Autism: explaining the enigma* by Uta Frith (Basil Blackwell, Oxford, 1989).

For a classic text of immense practical value, see *Autistic children: a guide for parents* by Lorna Wing (Constable, London, 1971).

For an overview of research into the 'theory of mind' hypothesis of autism (the view that in autism the social and communicative difficulties are the result of an inborn inability to understand other people's minds), see *Understanding other minds: perspectives from autism* by Simon Baron-Cohen, Helen Tager-Flusberg, and Donald Cohen (eds) (Oxford University Press, 1993).

The best account of different treatment approaches to autism that we know of is *The treatment of autistic children*, by Patricia Howlin and Michael Rutter (Wiley, Chichester, 1987).

Finally, an invaluable reference textbook on autism is the extensive *Handbook of autism and pervasive developmental disorders*, by Donald Cohen, Anne Donnellan, and Rhea Paul (Wiley, Chichester, 1987).

Glossary

Abnormalities of purine metabolism: The metabolic pathway that results in uric acid is termed the purine pathway. A number of enzyme deficiencies involved in this pathway may lead to developmental disorders, accompanied by autistic symptoms. The mechanisms in this are not well understood.

Asperger's syndrome: A condition with strong similarities to autism, but where the individual's early language development is not delayed, and may even be precocious. Language, however, is still used in a stilted and stereotyped manner. Intellectually, individuals with Asperger's syndrome usually function in the normal range of ability.

Attachment disorder: During normal child development there emerges (at around nine months of age) a set of 'attachment behaviours' that are earliest manifestations of a loving relationship between child and parent or care-giver. These behaviours include distress on separation and pleasure on reunion. In disorders of attachment the formation of this early relationship is disrupted or disturbed. This is particularly commonly seen in instances of child-abuse or neglect.

Atypical autism: A diagnosis reserved for those individuals who display the characteristic features of autism in two of the three key areas (language development, social development, and play development) but do not display the features in the third.

Behaviour therapy: Scientifically-based approach to modifying and shaping behaviour by identifying and manipulating the triggers and reinforcements of specific behaviours (see Appendix 3).

Biedl–Bardet syndrome: Also called Lawrence–Moon–Biedl syndrome. A syndrome of obesity, pigmentation of the retina, and extra digits, accompanied by mental handicap.

Brain stem: A term referring to a part of the brain that extends from the spinal cord to the mid-brain. It includes the medulla.

CAT scans: CAT stands for Computed Axial Tomography. This is an advanced form of X-ray which is especially useful for obtaining pictures of the brain.

Chromosome: The structure housing the genetic material and genes responsible for the inheritance of many (but not all) physical and mental characteristics.

Coffin-Siris syndrome: A syndrome of congenital abnormalities, including growth deficiencies, microcephaly (small head), excessive body hair, and joint laxity, coupled with mental handicap.

Congenital anomaly syndromes: A collective term for disorders of physical development during the fetal period.

Congenital cytomegalovirus: A condition resulting from intrauterine infection with the cytomegalovirus.

Congenital rubella: A condition resulting from intra-uterine infection with the rubella (German measles) virus.

Cornelia de Lange syndrome: A congenital anomaly syndrome characterized by mental retardation, unusual facial appearance, and small hands and feet, sometimes accompanied by epilepsy.

Cytomegalovirus: A virus that may produce a 'flu'-like illness in adults, but which if it infects a pregnant mother (particularly in the early stages of pregnancy) may damage the development of the unborn baby and lead to mental handicap and physical disabilities.

Deixis: A part of communication in which the meaning of a word or gesture depends on the particular context at the time (for example, the words 'here' or 'there').

Developmental receptive language disorder: A disorder characterized by a difficulty in understanding speech and language.

Disintegrative disorder: A condition where regression and loss of skills follow a period of normal development. Initially, there may be a period of anxiety and confusion, which is followed by intellectual and behavioural decline. Bladder and bowel control may also be lost. Sometimes the 'disintegration' is due to rare neurological diseases.

Dizygotic twins: Twin pregnancies resulting from the fertilization of two eggs. Consequently the twins are genetically related in the same way as most other siblings are.

EEG: Electroencephalogram. This is a procedure for measuring the brain's electrical activity. It involves simply sticking wires to the scalp and recording the natural activity of the brain.

Echolalia: A term referring to the repetition of words or phrases. Echolalia may occur immediately after the phrases have been said, or may be delayed and occur some time later.

Elective mutism: A disorder characterized by mutism in specific situations (i.e. the child speaks only in certain circumstances). Often there is evidence of extreme shyness and sensitivity.

Epilepsy: A group of conditions resulting from abnormal electrical discharges in the brain which can produce seizures and disturbances in consciousness.

Event-related potential: Refers to the measurable electrical activity in the brain following stimulation.

Fragile X syndrome: An inherited chromosomal abnormality that leads to learning difficulties and mental handicap. So called because the X chromosome possesses a site of fragility.

Frontal lobes: The front parts of the cerebral hemispheres of the brain, responsible for many higher cognitive functions (complex reasoning, planning, etc.).

Herpes encephalitis: A brain infection resulting from a type of herpes virus (different from the herpes virus responsible for the sexually transmitted disease herpes). The brain infection often damages the regions of the brain responsible for memory.

Histidinaemia: A term that refers to an elevated level of histidine (an amino acid) in the blood. It is usually benign, but has been reported in conjunction with autism.

Holding therapy: A controversial treatment advocated for autism. It entails physically forcing the child to hold and look at the parents.

Hyperactivity: A term used to refer to a syndrome of over-activity, inattentiveness, and impulsivity. The hyperactivity has to occur across a number of different situations for it to be significantly abnormal.

Hyperkinetic disorder with stereotypies: Extreme hyperactivity coupled with stereotyped and repetitive behaviour.

IQ: Intelligence Quotient. This is a measure of intellectual ability derived from the administration of standardized tests of different aspects of cognition and language.

Leber's amaurosis: A form of blindness.

Limbic system: A group of interlinked brain structures which are responsible for aspects of emotional, sexual, and eating behaviour.

Mental handicap: A syndrome comprising impaired intelligence and learning difficulties. By itself this term does not indicate the cause of these problems, and different subgroups of mental handicap, caused by different factors, exist.

Moebius' syndrome: A congenial anomaly syndrome characterized by abnormalities in the nerve-supply to eye muscles and groups of facial muscles. This results in paralysis of certain facial muscles.

Monozygotic twins: Twins that derive from only one fertilized egg. After a number of cell divisions new cells are split to form the two fetuses. They are genetically identical.

MRI scans: Magnetic Resonance Imaging scans. A relatively newly developed form of imaging. It entails the measurement of the particles emitted from the body after exposure to a large fluctuating magnetic force.

Neologisms: Made-up words not belonging to any conventional vocabulary, but not meaningless.

Neurofibromatosis (von Recklinghausen's disease): An inherited genetic disorder, which can take the form of producing coffee-like skin marks and abnormalities of the nerves.

Noonan syndrome: A syndrome of multiple physical anomalies, including heart, chest, and facial abnormalities, accompanied by mental handicap.

Obsession: A repetitive, unwanted irrational thought, often leading to compulsive behaviour.

PET and SPET scans: PET stands for Positron Emission Tomography. This type of scan involves the administration of radio-labelled substances (breathing special gases, injections, etc.) which are preferentially taken up by certain regions of the brain or body, and then emit radio signals from them. These signals are measured with a scanner, and the information is used to create a picture of the region under investigation. This is similar to SPET (Single Photon Emission Tomography), but produces a more accurate image. SPET is however more widely available, and so is often recommended in preference to PET.

Phenylketonuria: An inherited biochemical abnormality that results in faulty breakdown of key substances in the blood. Consequently there are phenylketones in the urine (hence the name 'phenylketonuria'), and an accumulation of noxious substances which may damage the brain. A special diet can prevent problems.

Pica: The eating and chewing of inedible substances.

Pronoun reversal: The incorrect use of words like 'you'.

Retinoblastoma: A tumour of the retina of the eye, often evident in infancy.

Rett's syndrome: A condition affecting females, characterized by profound handicap, spasticity in the legs, and problems with walking, as well as a tendency to hand-washing or hand-wringing repetitive movements.

Rubella: The rubella virus is responsible for German measles. If a pregnant mother develops German measles, the virus may, as with the cytomegalovirus, also infect and damage the unborn baby. An infant that has been infected by rubella may as a result be blind and/or deaf, and have additional mental handicap.

Savant abilities: A condition in which special talents exist in individuals with otherwise moderate or profound mental handicap. The talents tend to be in the areas of music, calendrical calculation, maths, or drawing. Such an individual may also be known as an *idiot savant*, or autistic savant. Many savants also have autism.

Specific language delay: A condition in which language is delayed in development.

Stereotypy: Repetitive behaviour, often of the hands or fingers.

Tuberous sclerosis: An inherited genetic disorder that produces growths in the brain and peripheral nervous system and special skin blemishes.

Williams syndrome: A syndrome of infantile hyper-calcaemia (elevated blood-calcium levels), heart abnormalities, and a characteristic facial appearance. As yet, the cause of the syndrome is unknown.

Index